नागः आरण्ये

नागः आरण्ये

Serpent in the Wilderness

Andy Richter

KEHRER

Like the rays of the moon
the light of yoga is expanding.
All religions, beliefs and sects
are receiving shelter
under the kalpataru of yoga.
Towards the evolution of consciousness
yoga has done unforgettable work.
Yoga will become tomorrow's culture
and will show
a new way of life for mankind.

Sri Swami Satyananda Saraswati

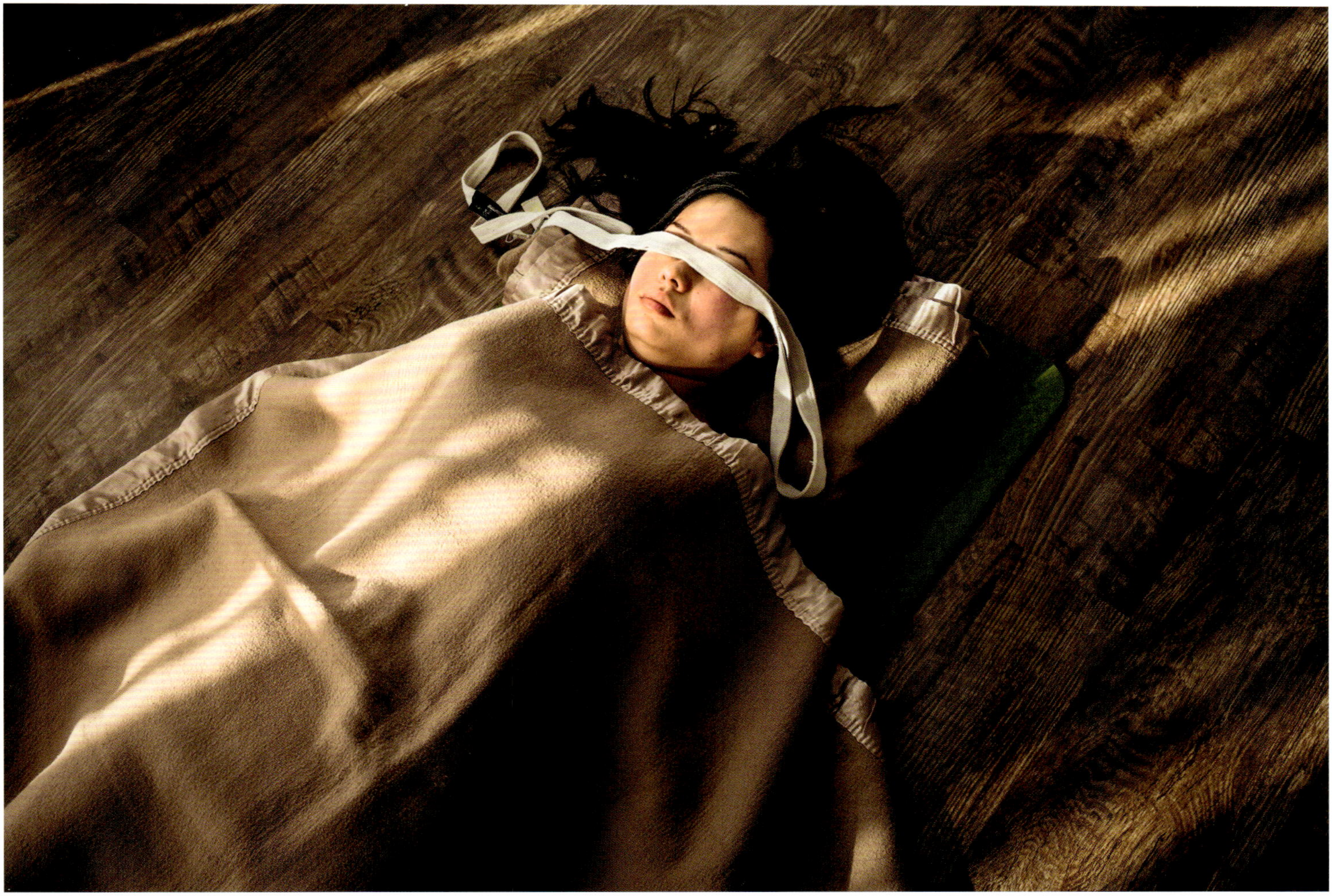

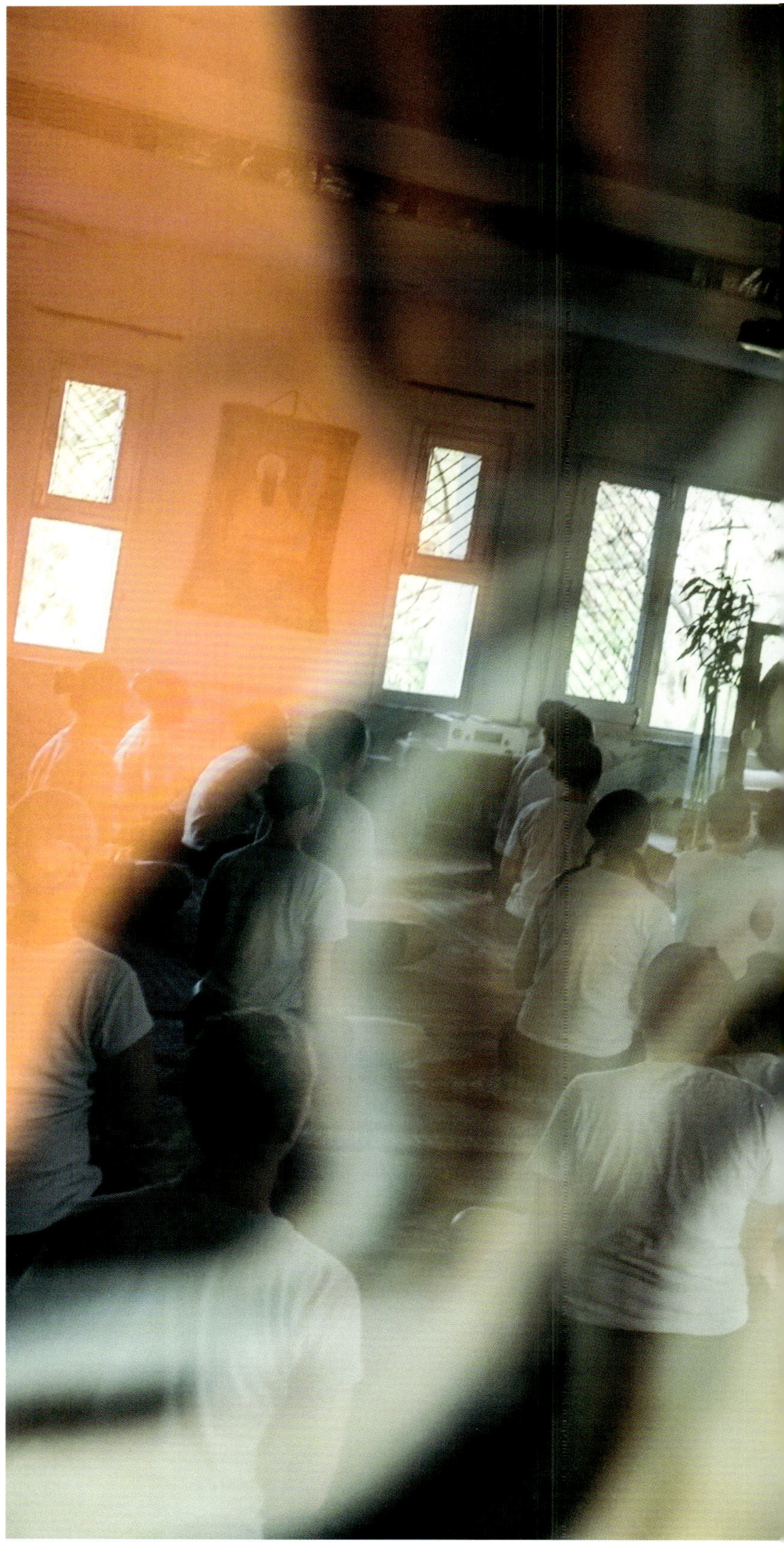

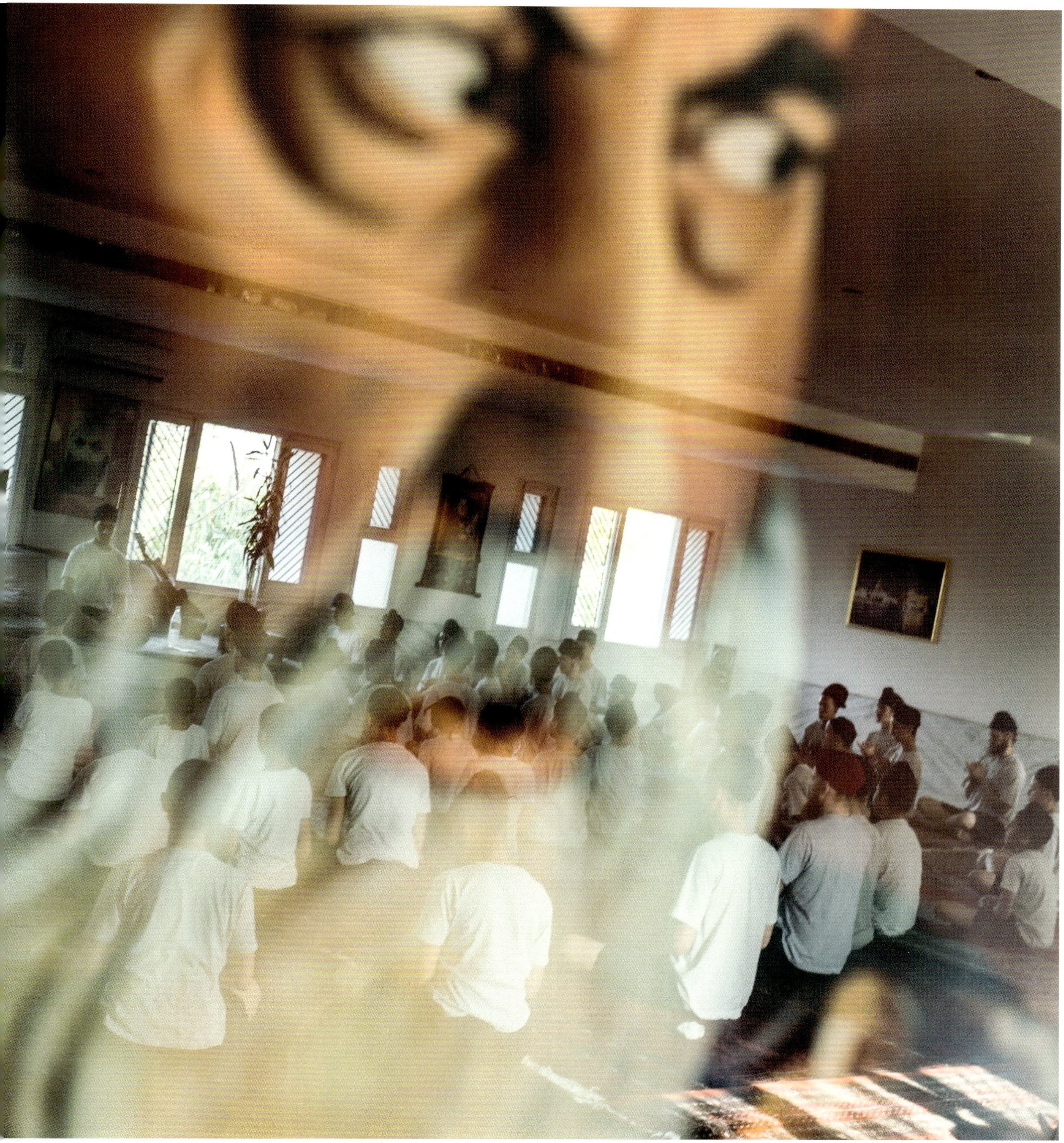

Travel light,
live light,
spread the light,
be the light.

Yogi Bhajan

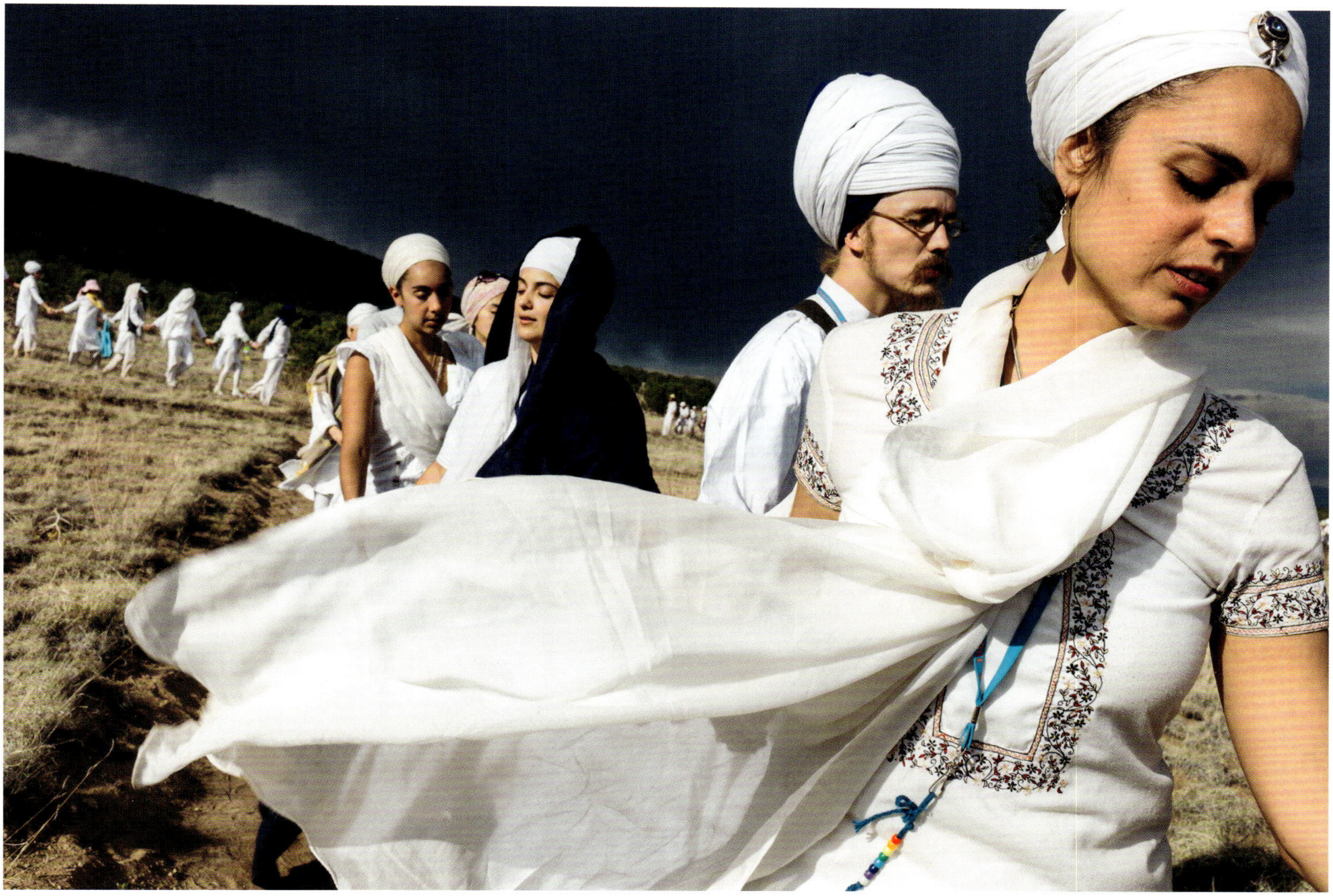

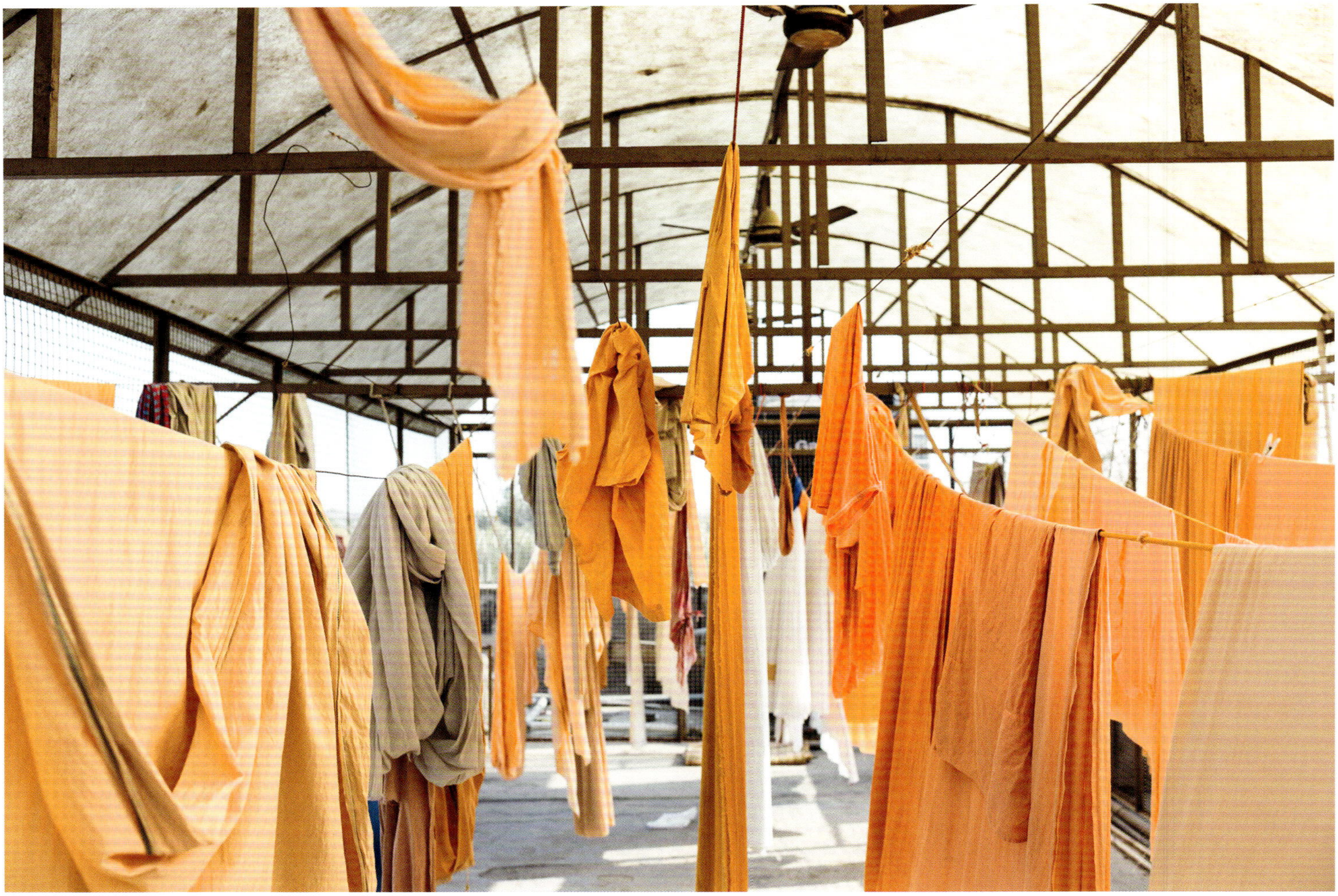

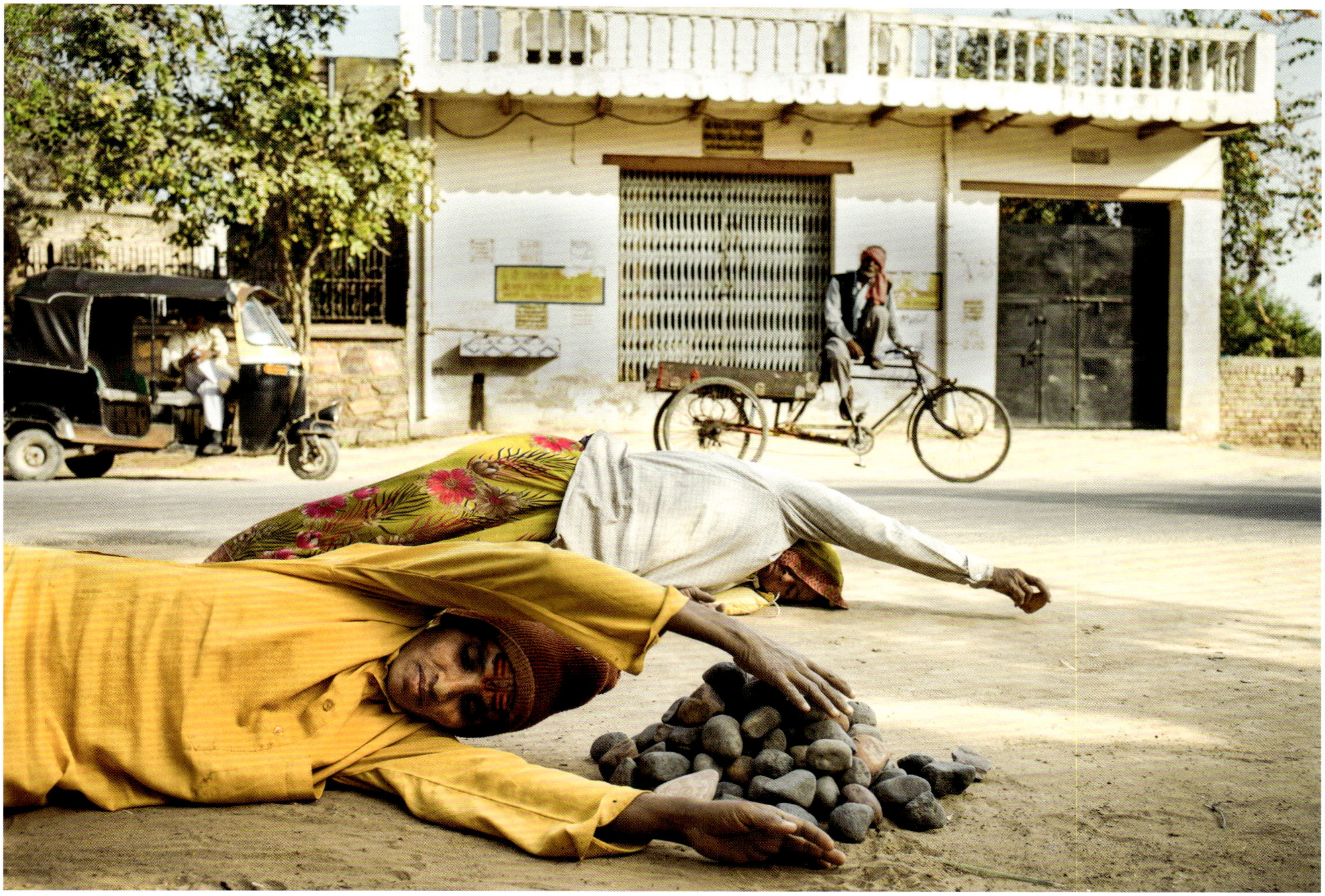

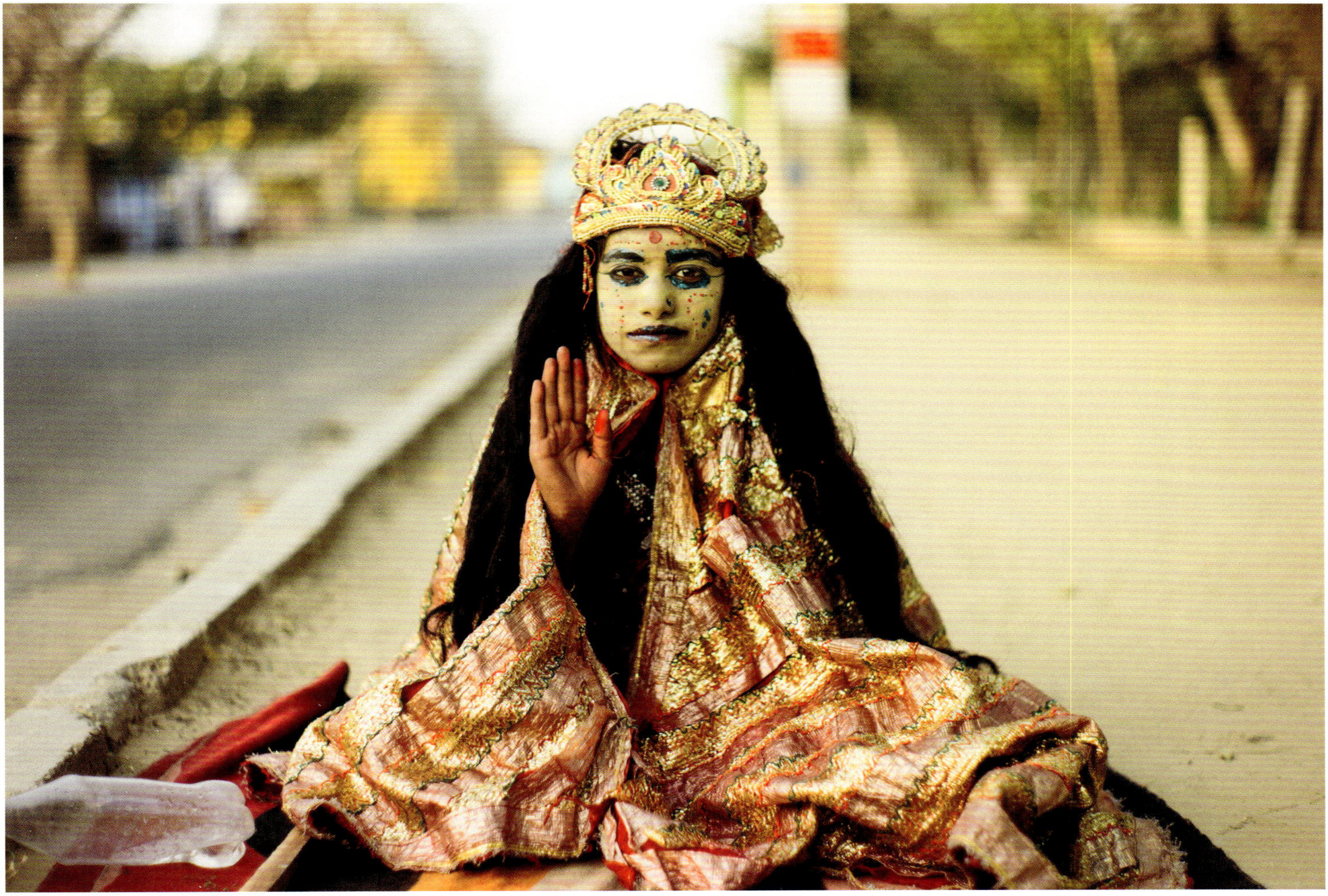

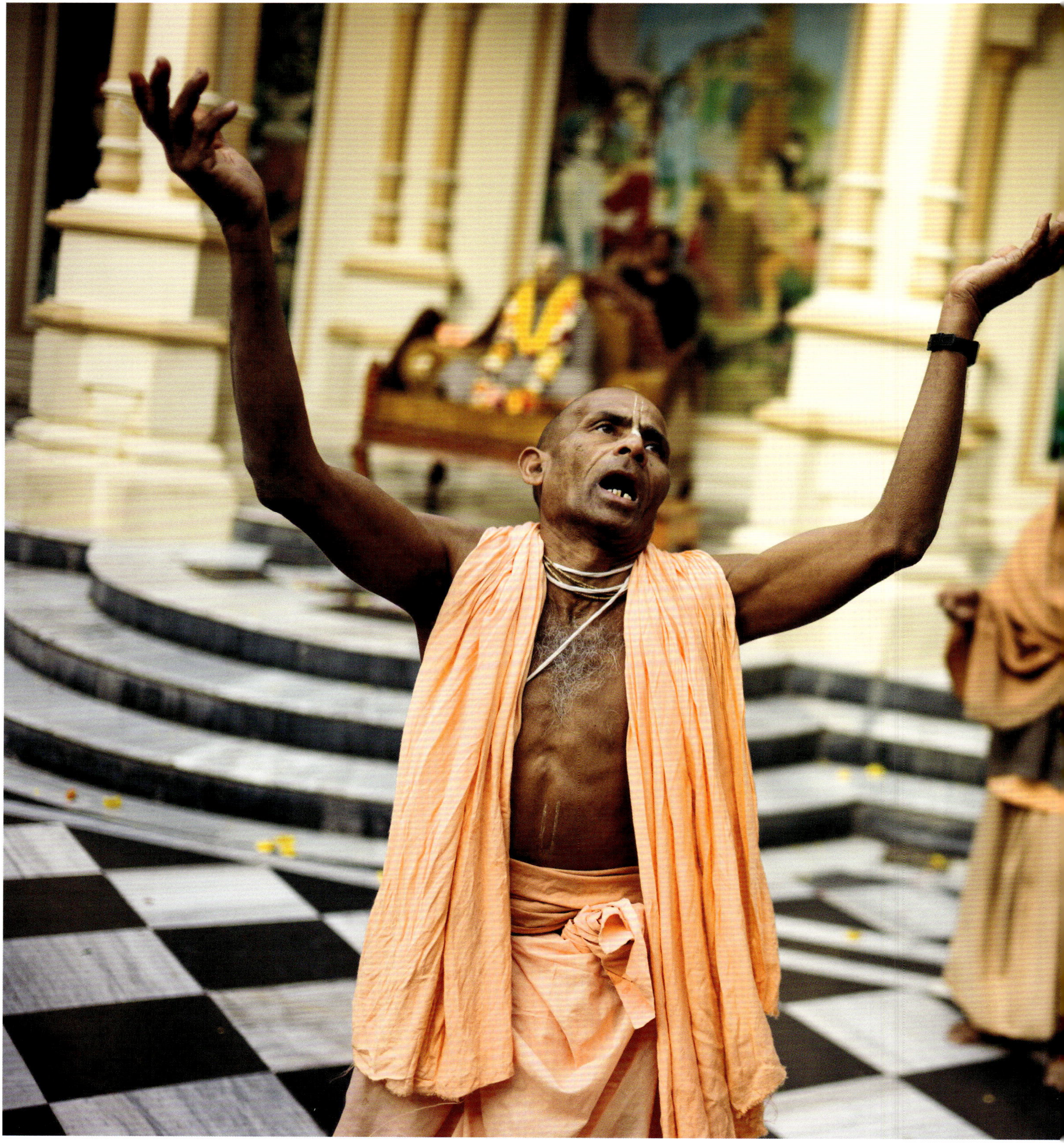

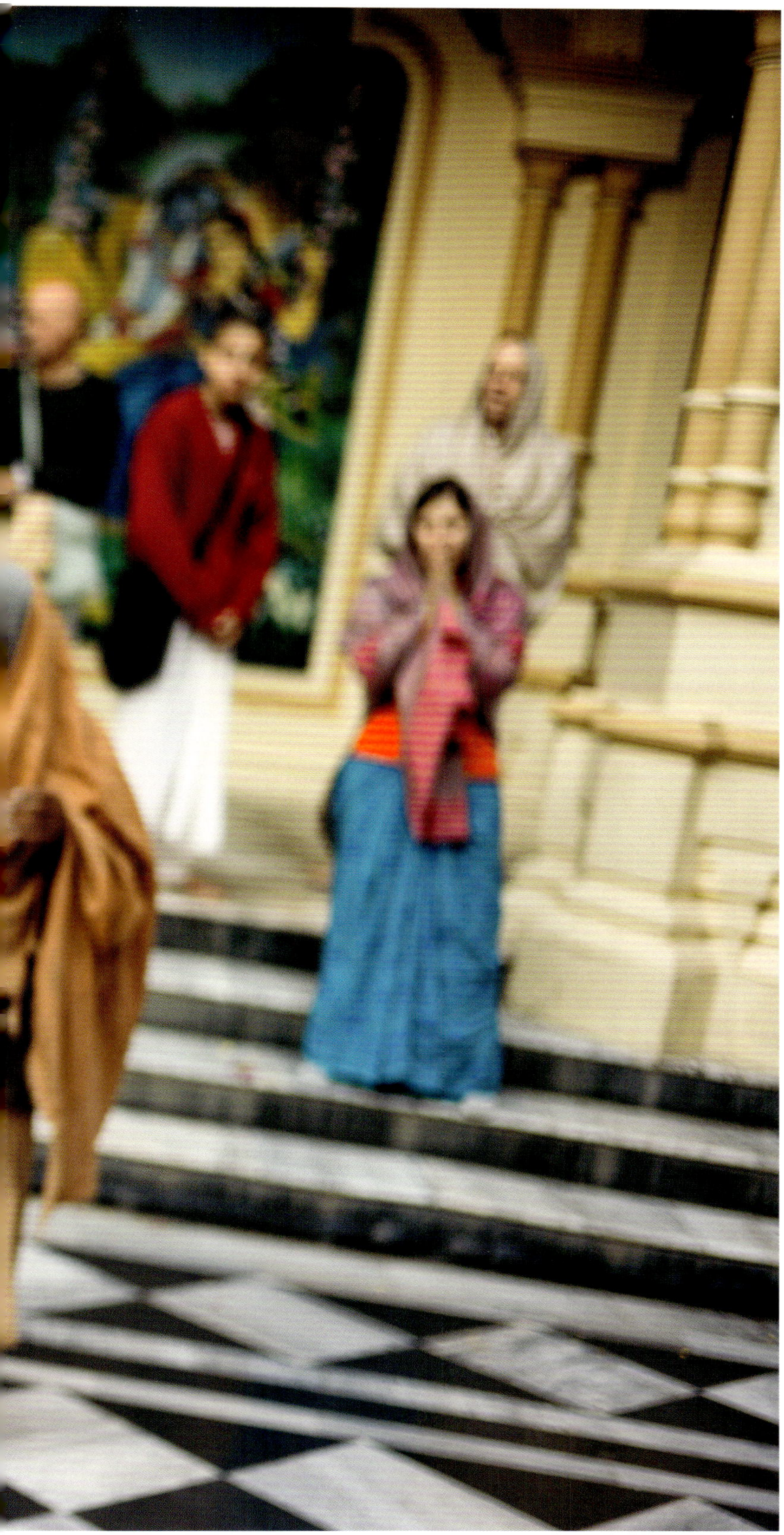

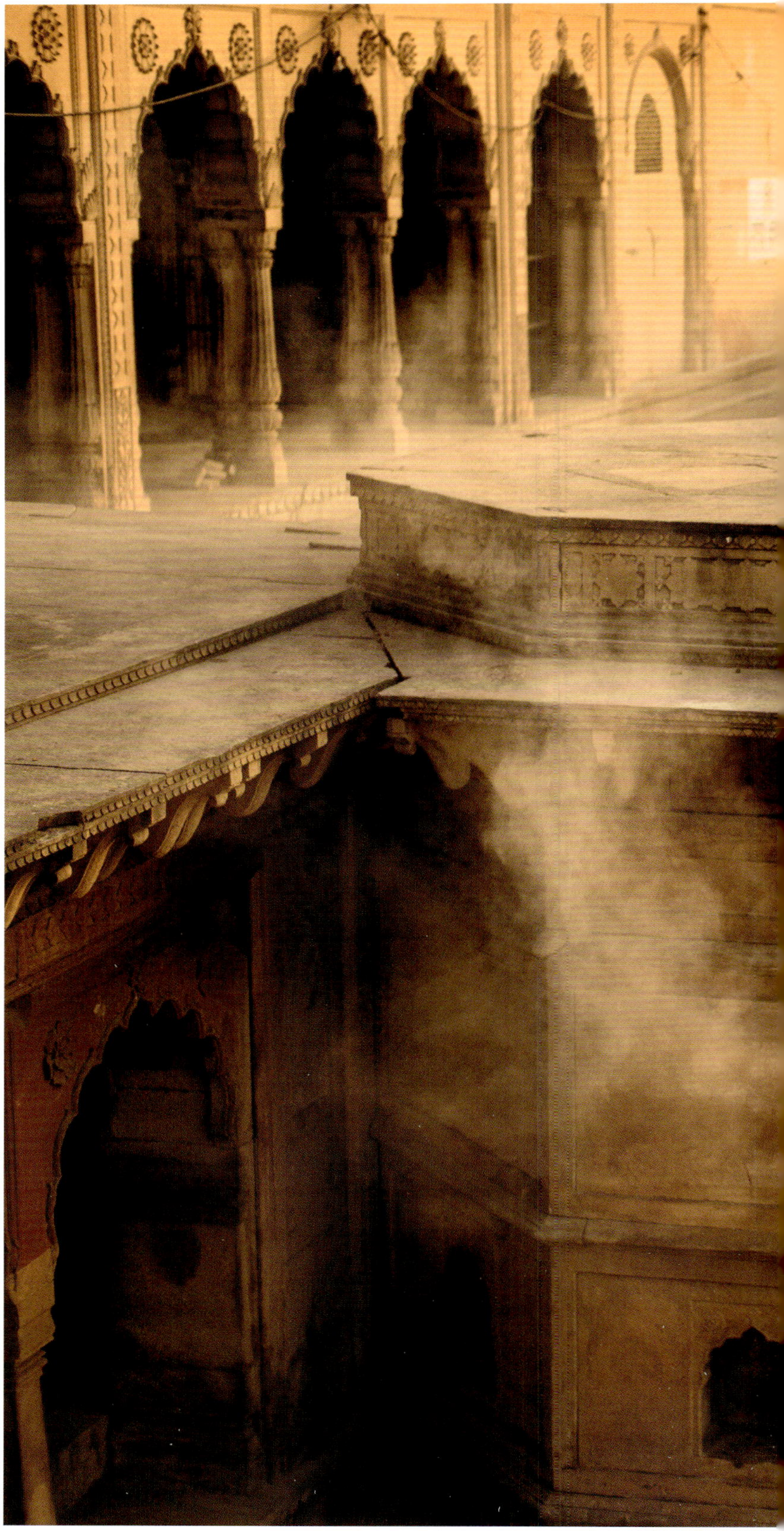

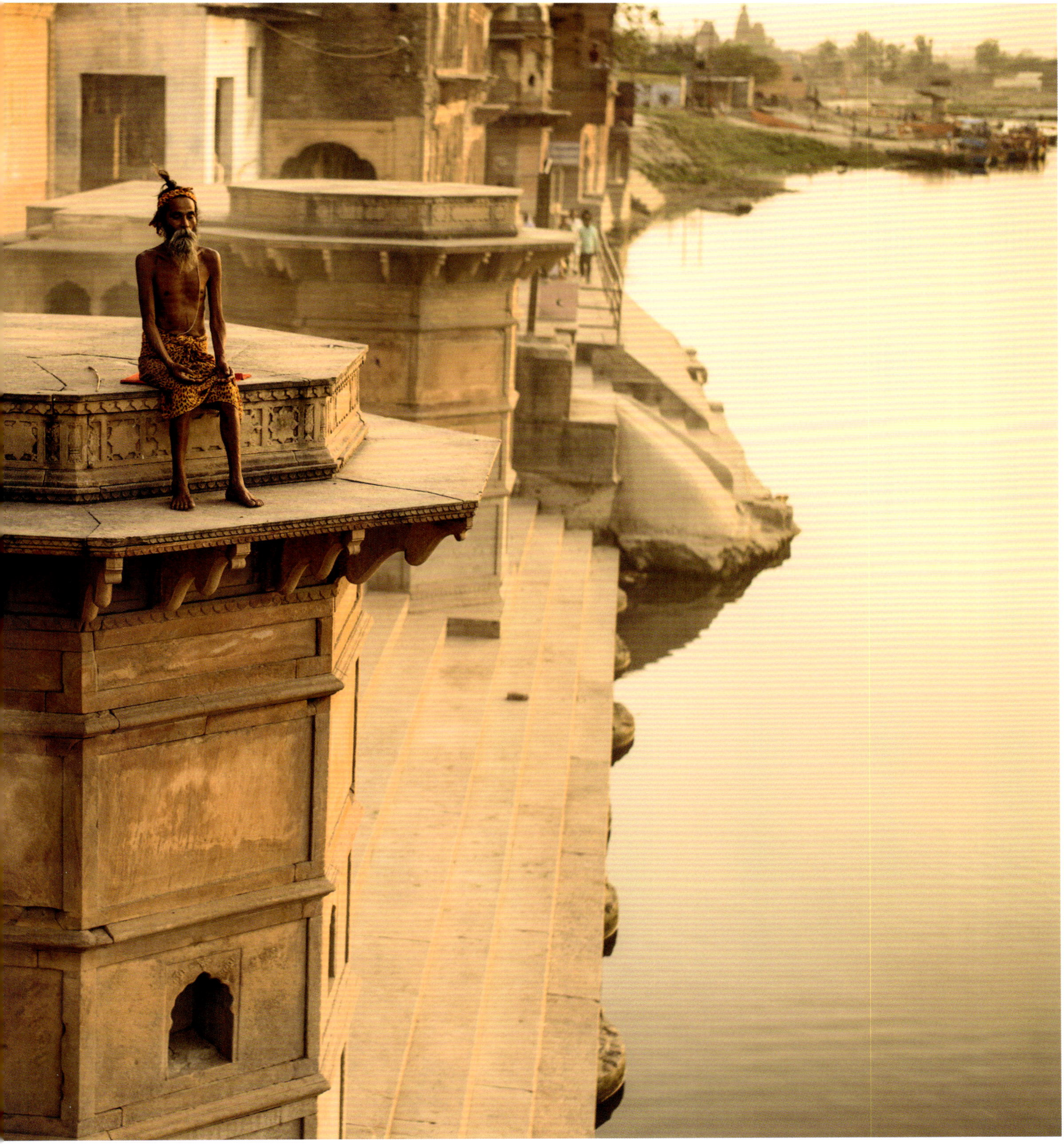

Yoga allows you to find
a new kind of freedom
that you may not have known
even existed.

B.K.S. Iyengar

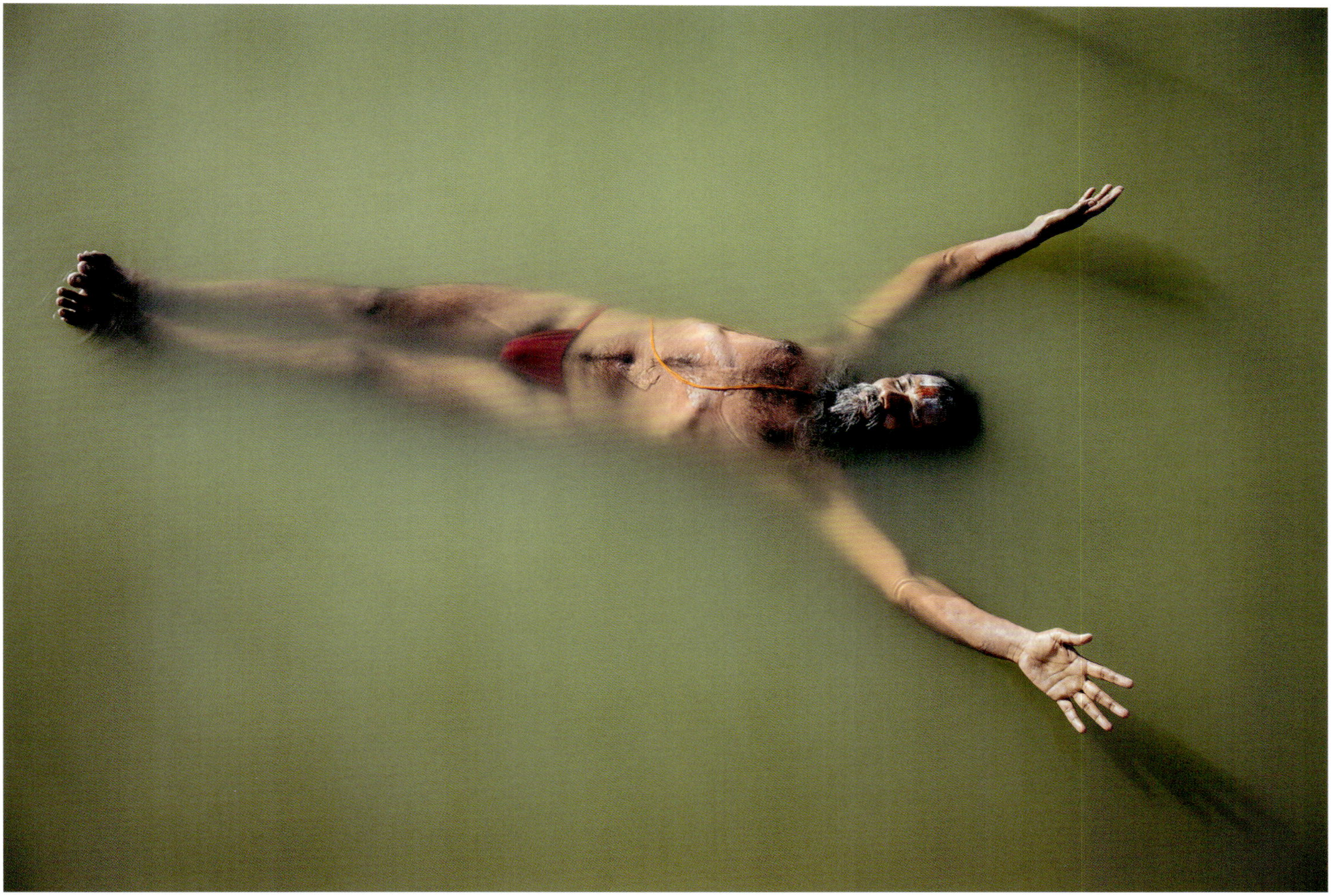

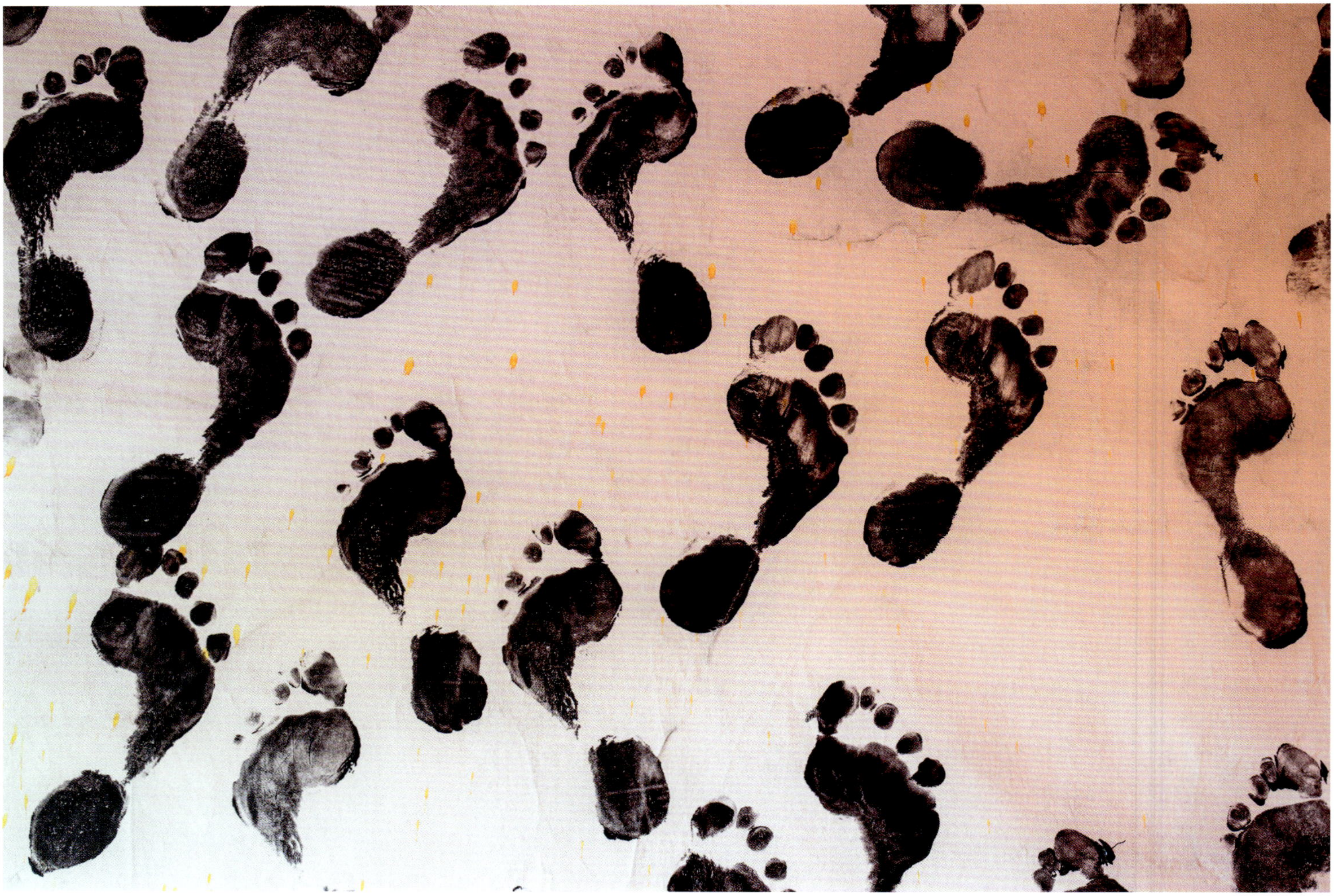

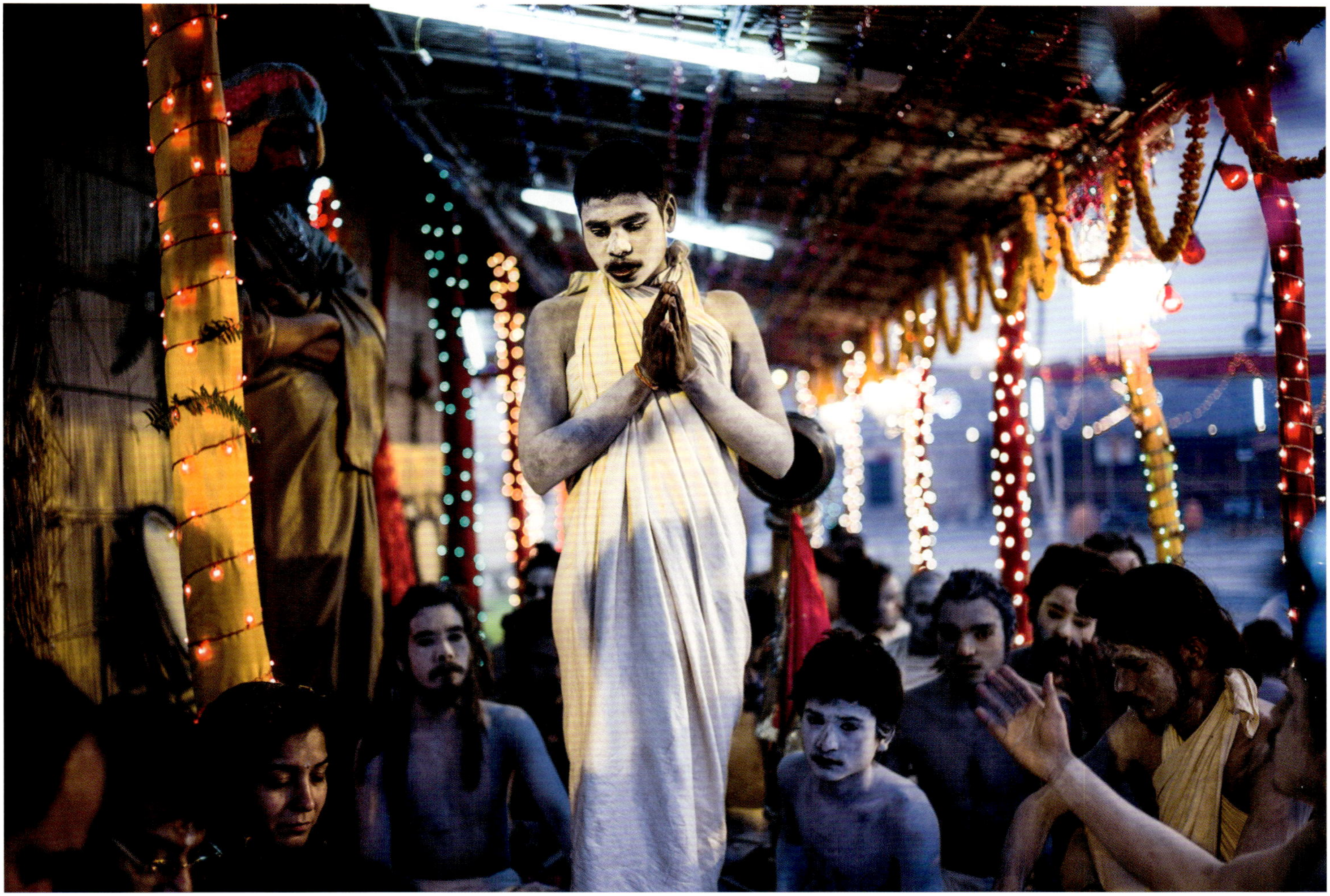

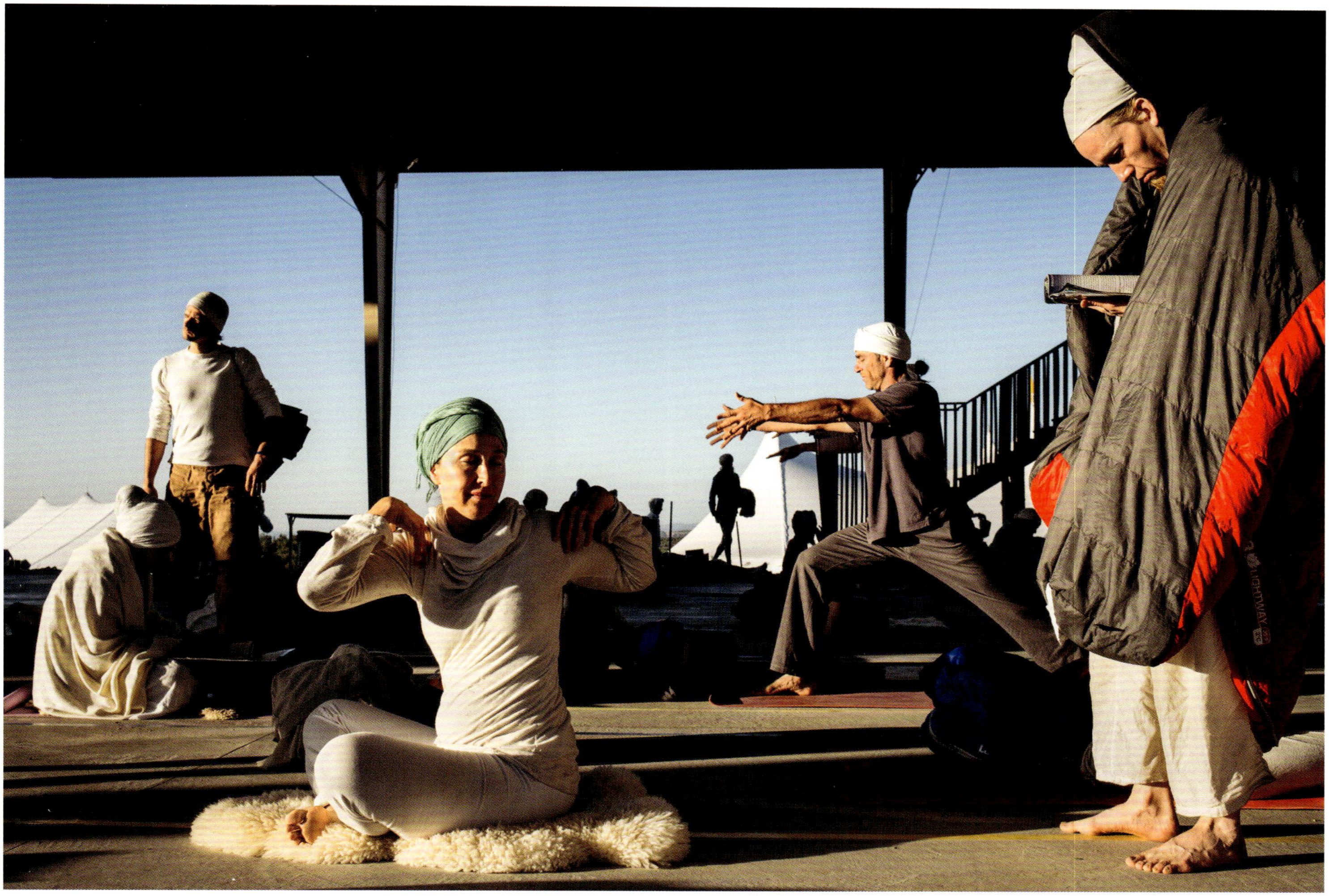

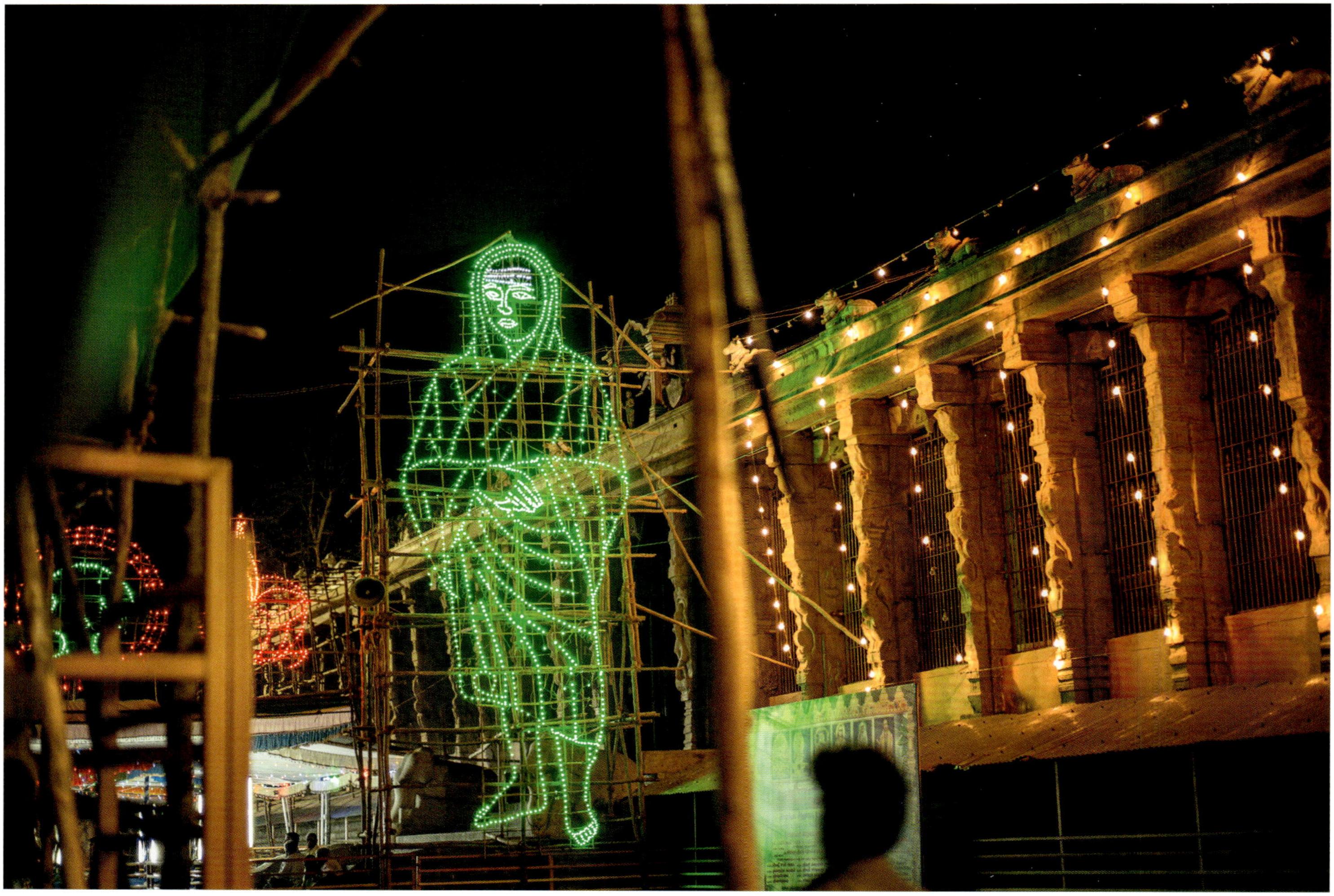

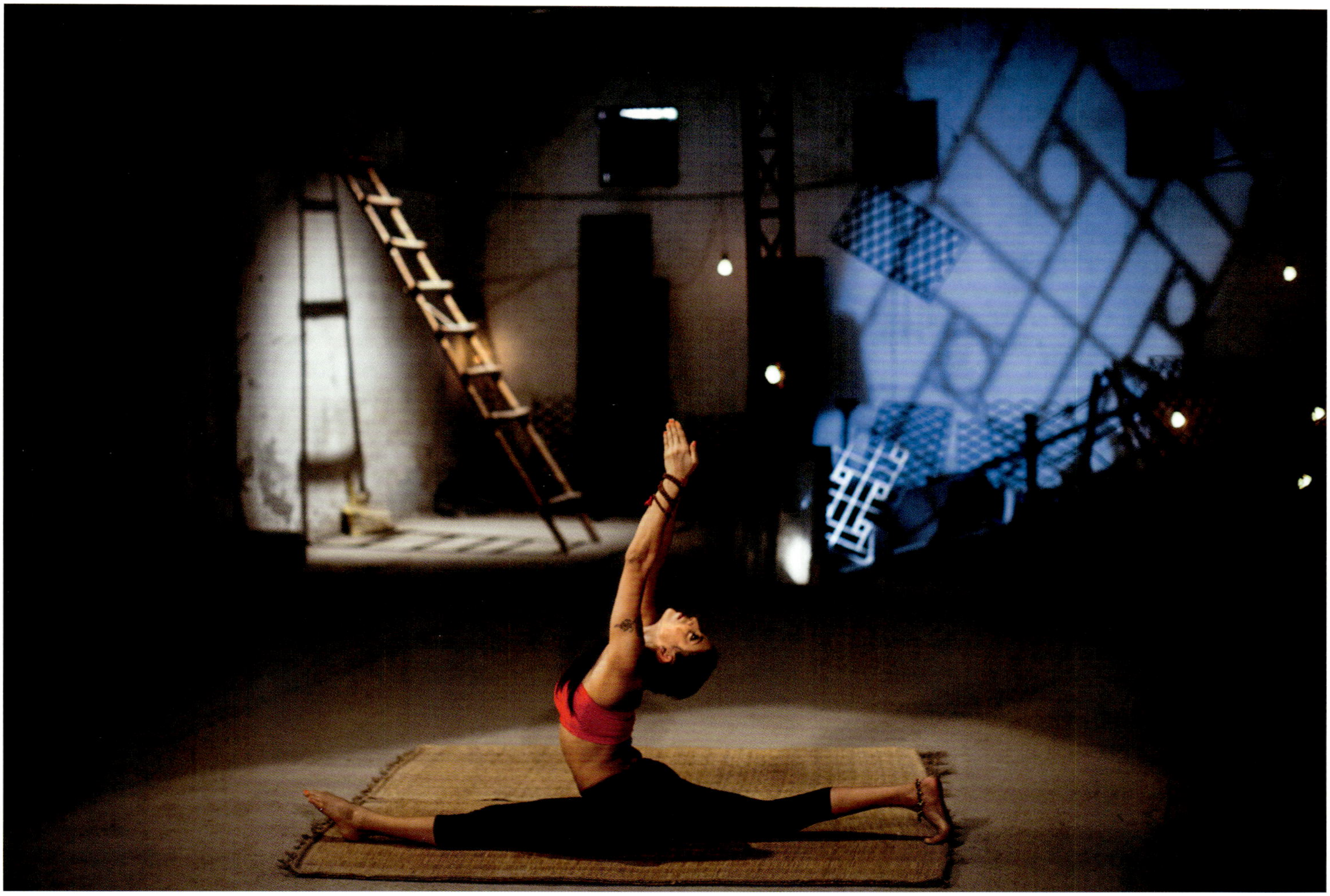

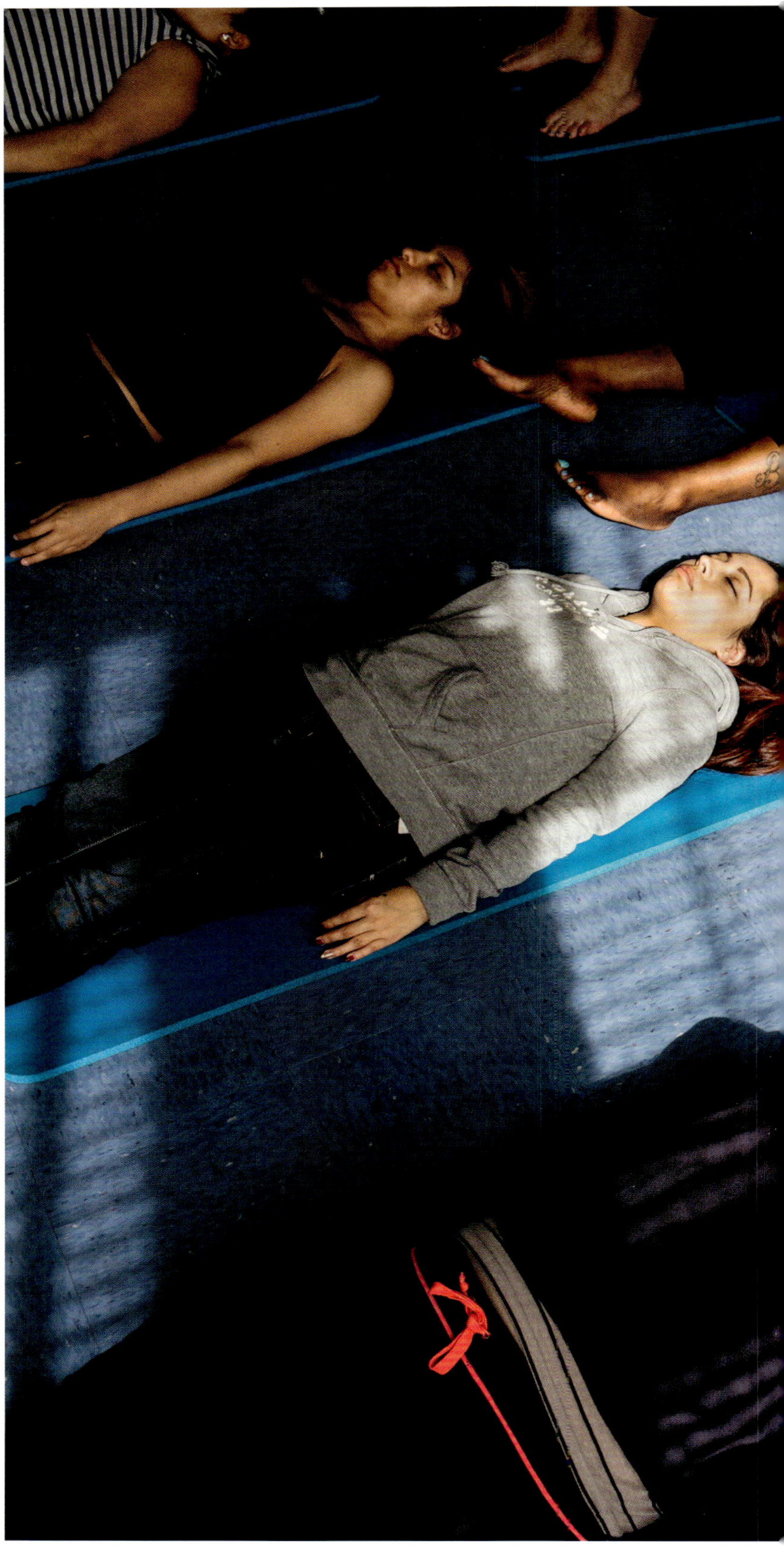

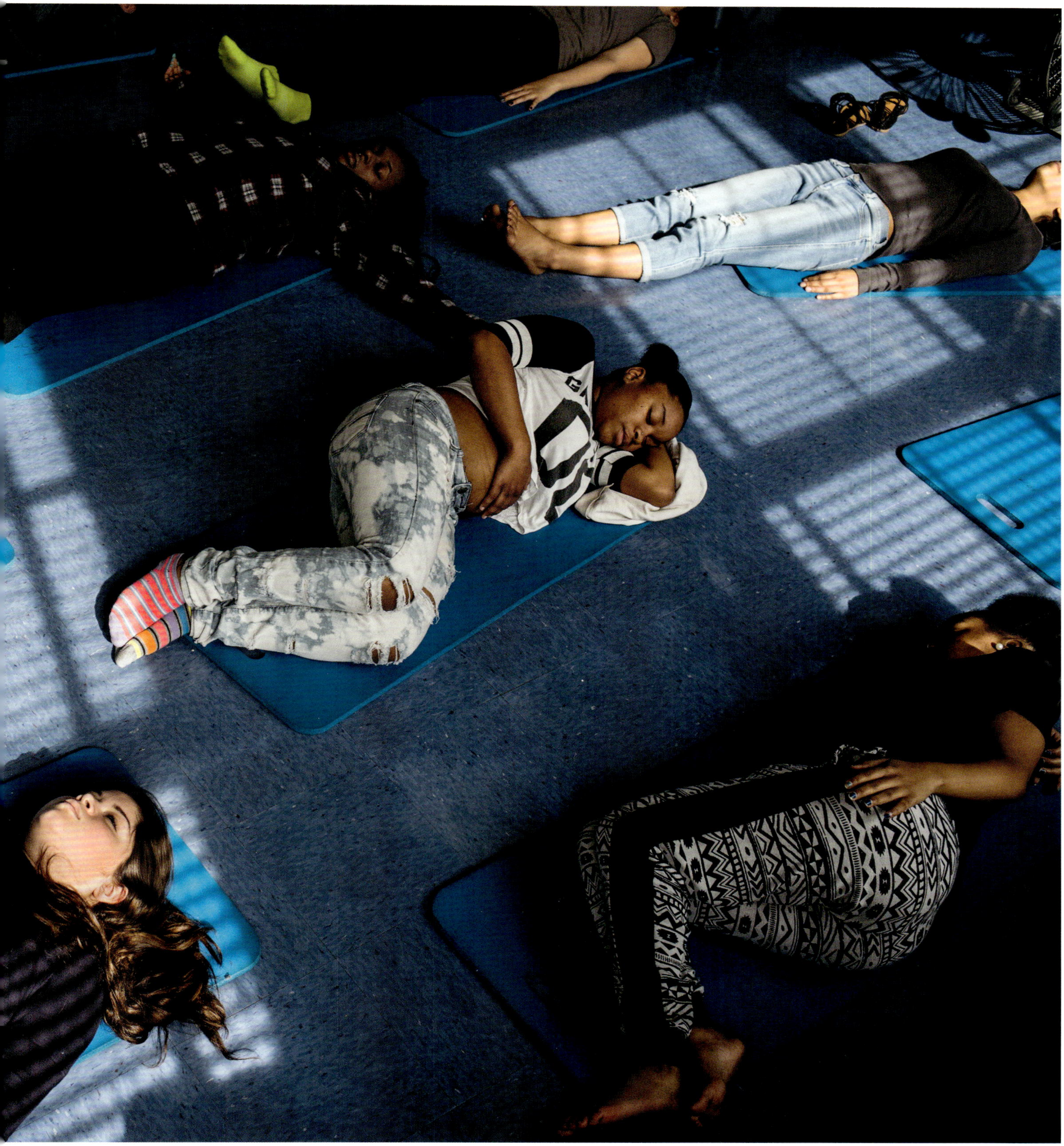

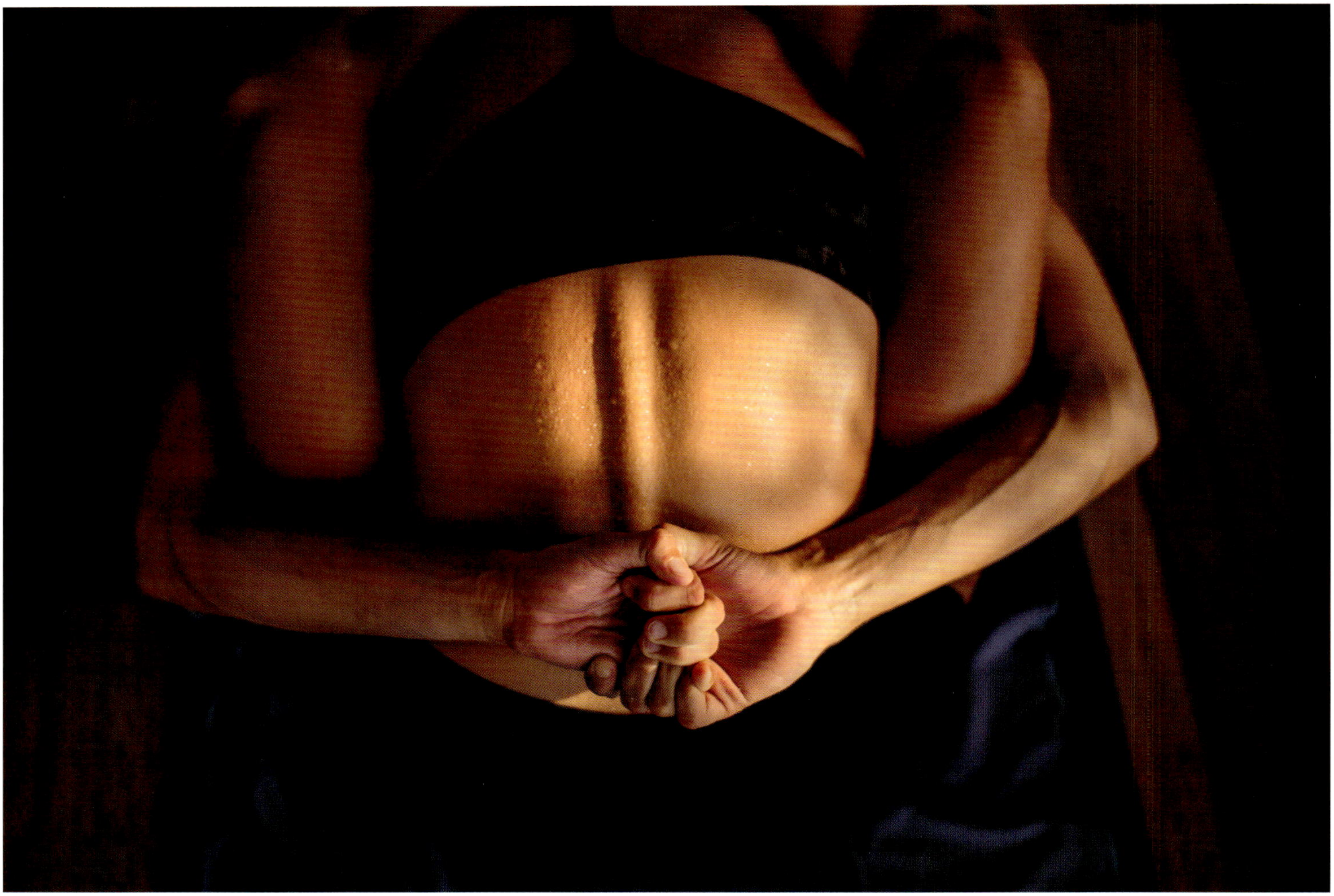

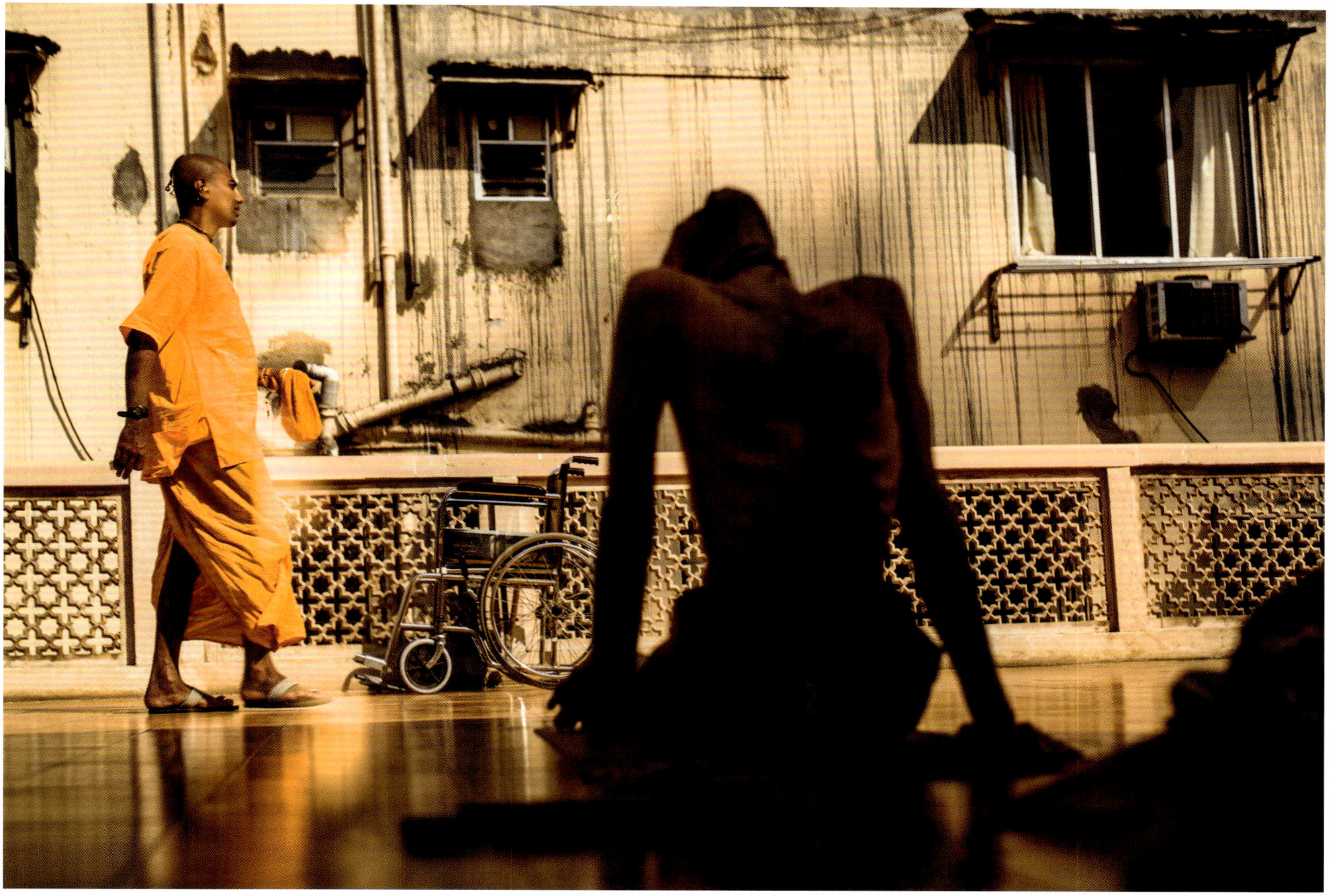

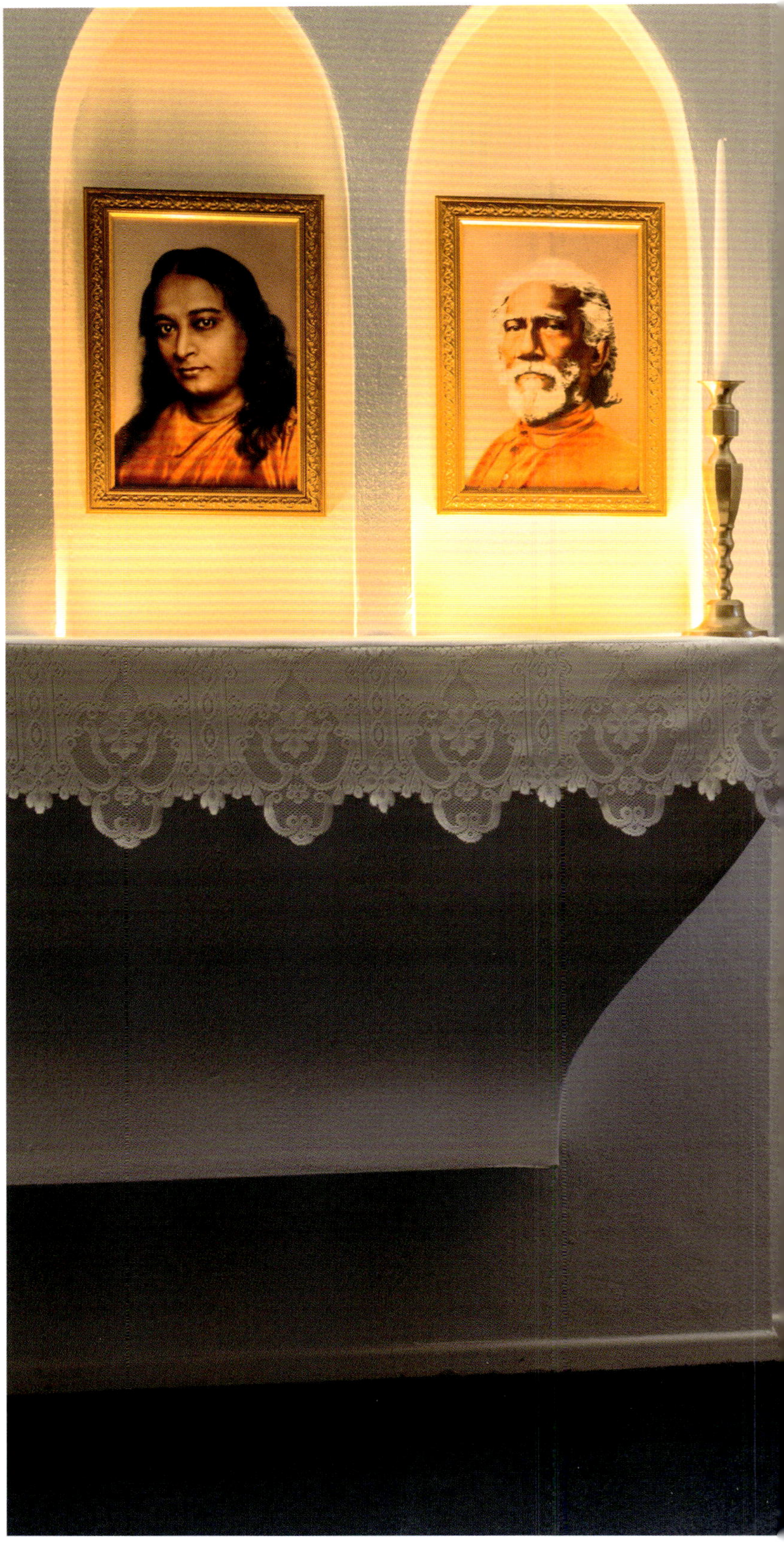

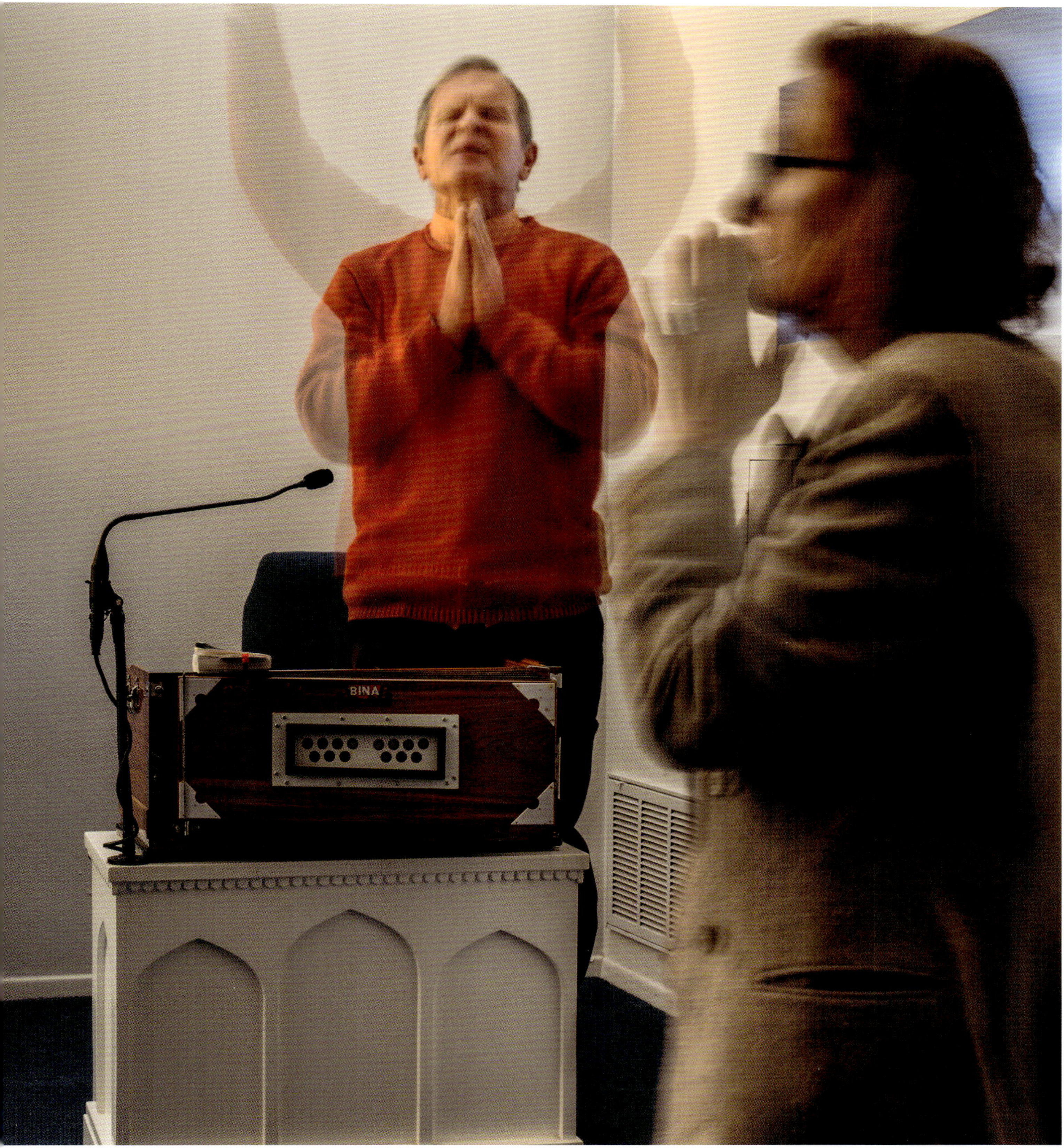
BINA

It is not necessary to meet
your guru on the physical plane.
The guru is not external.

Neem Karoli Baba

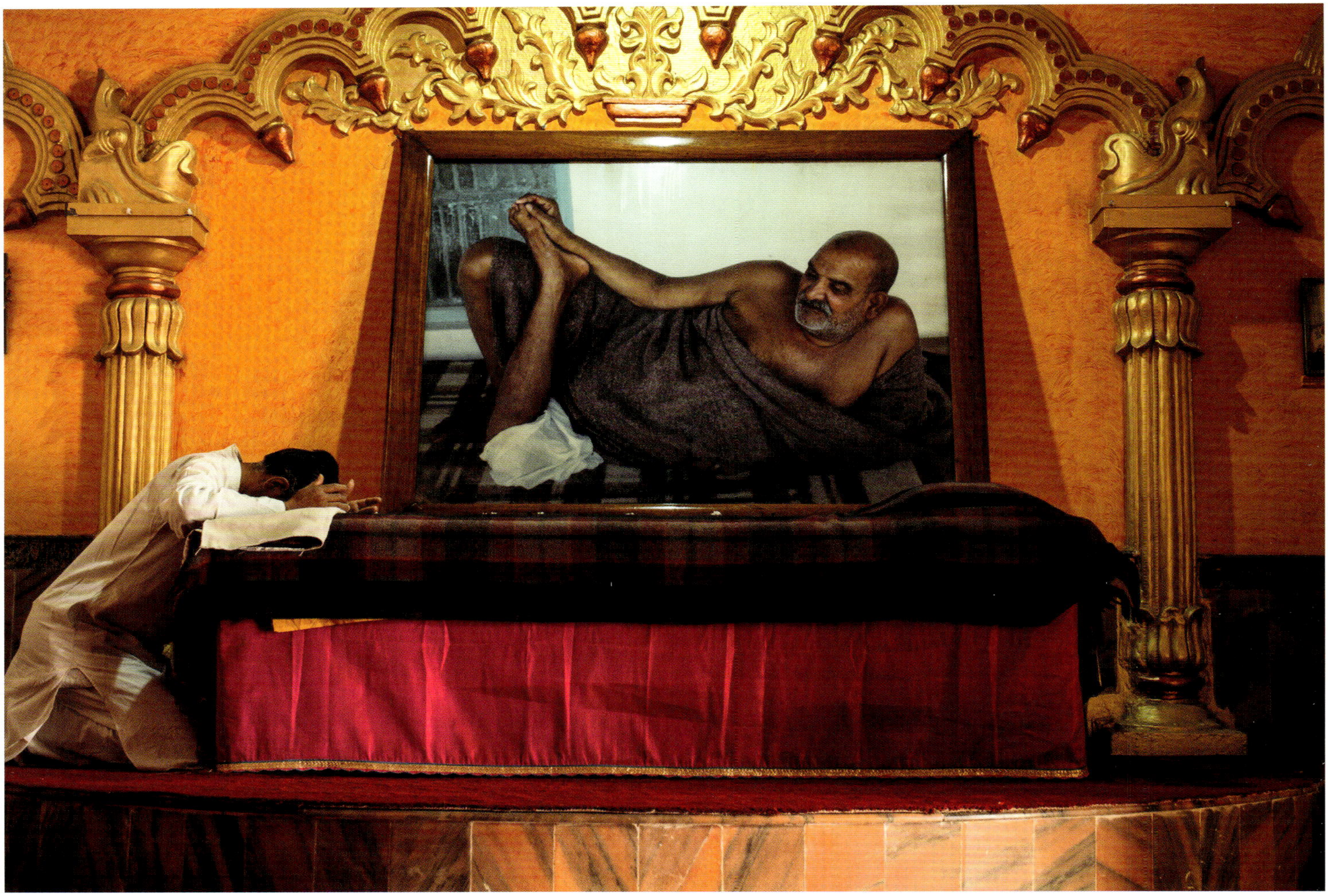

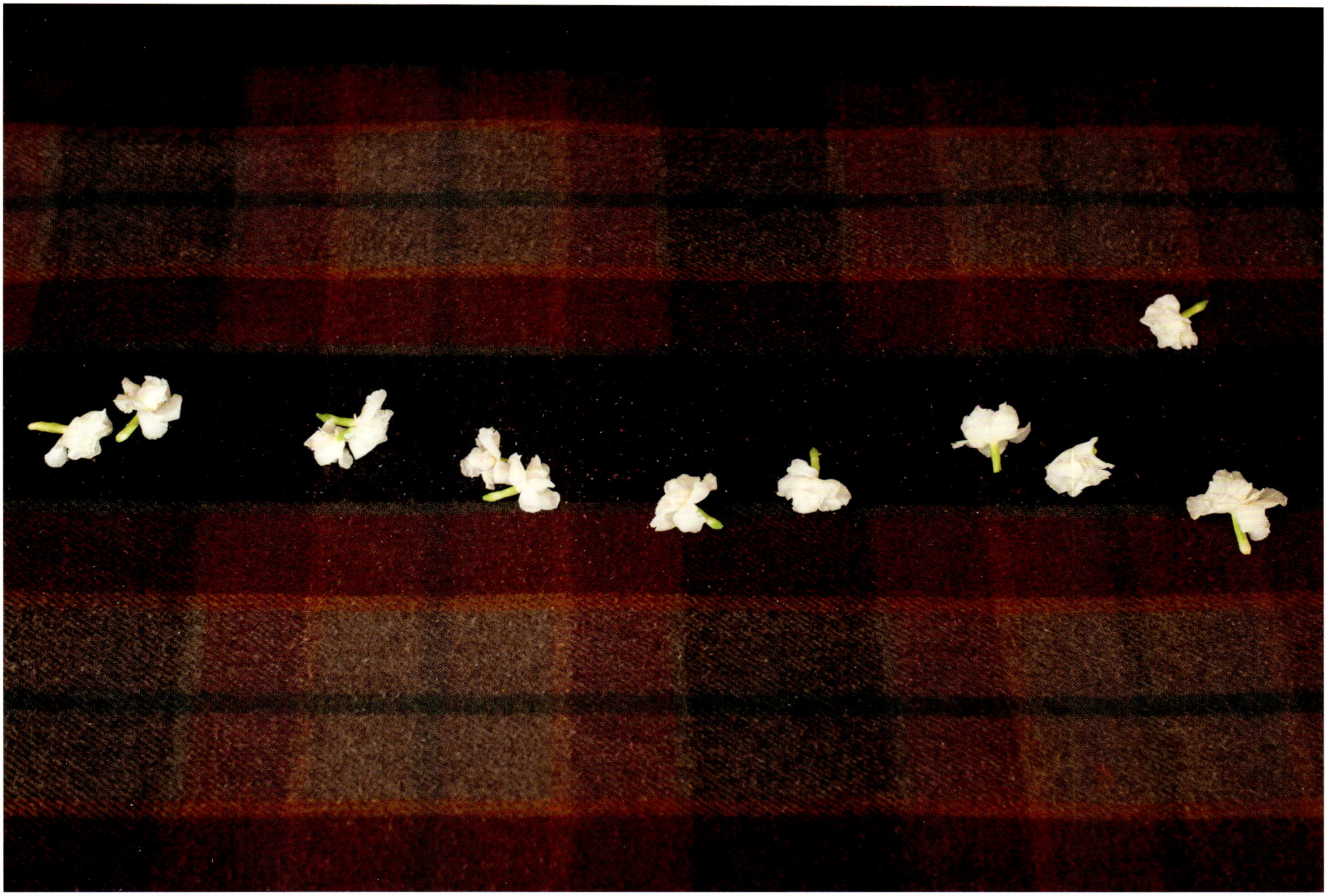

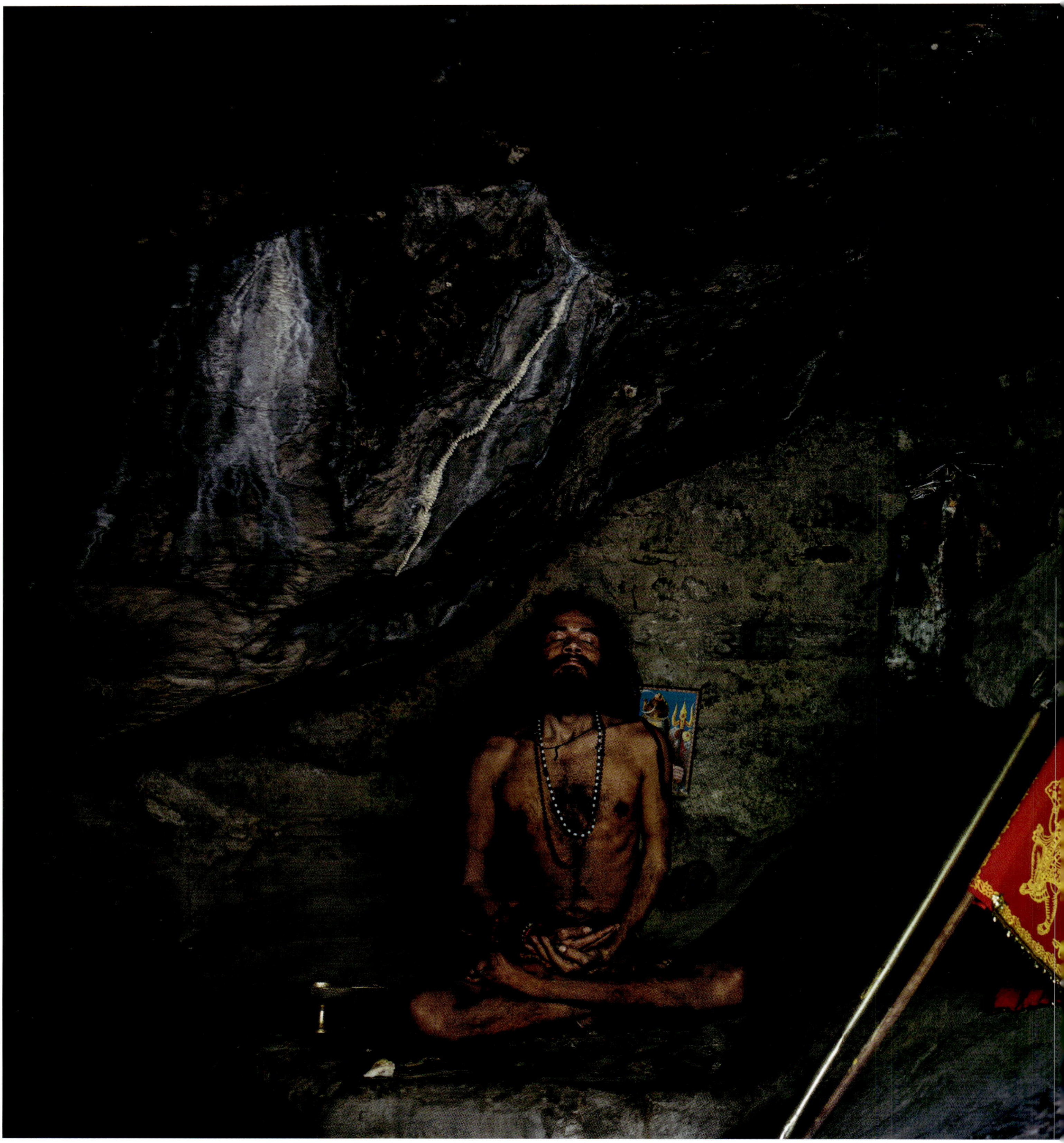

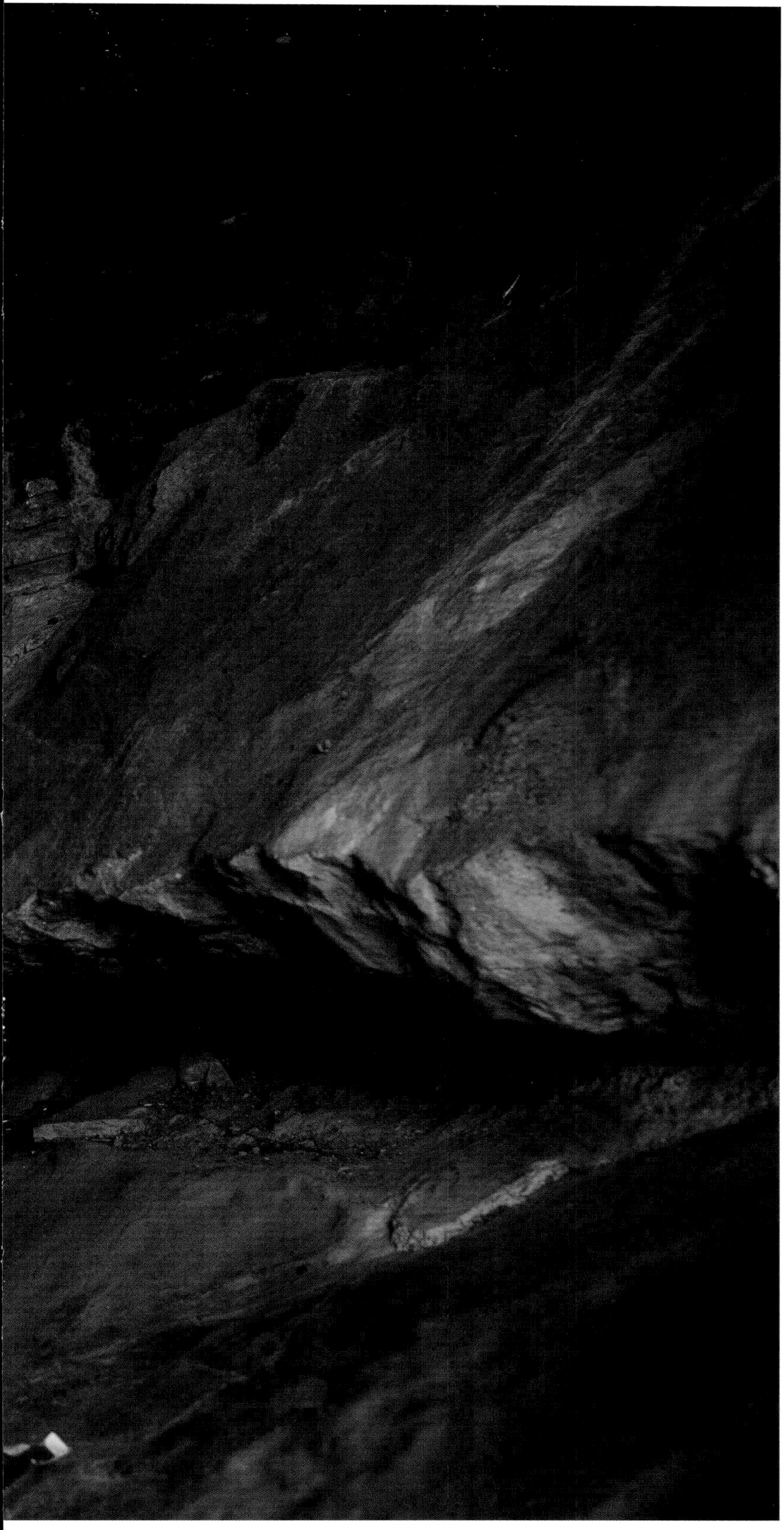

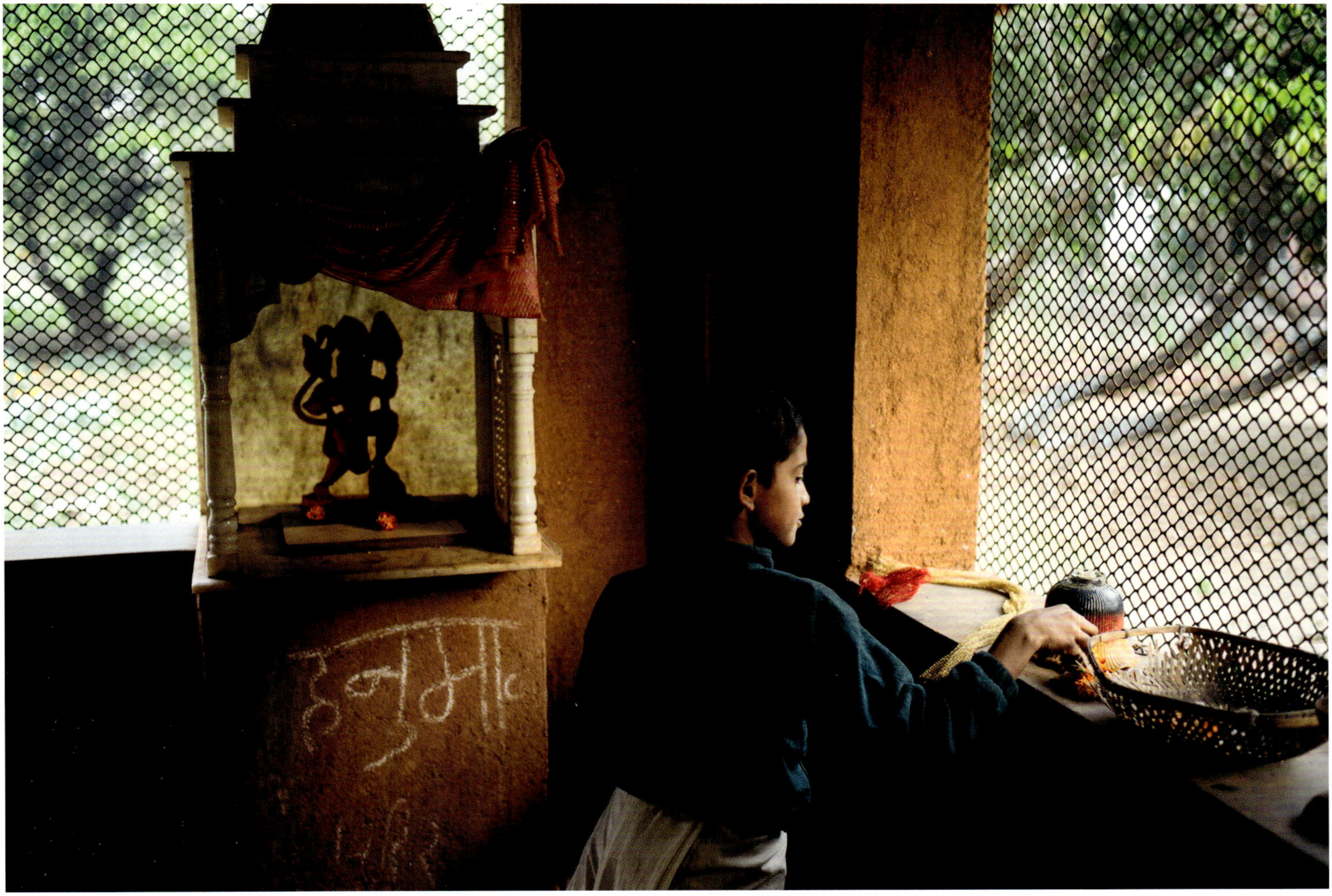

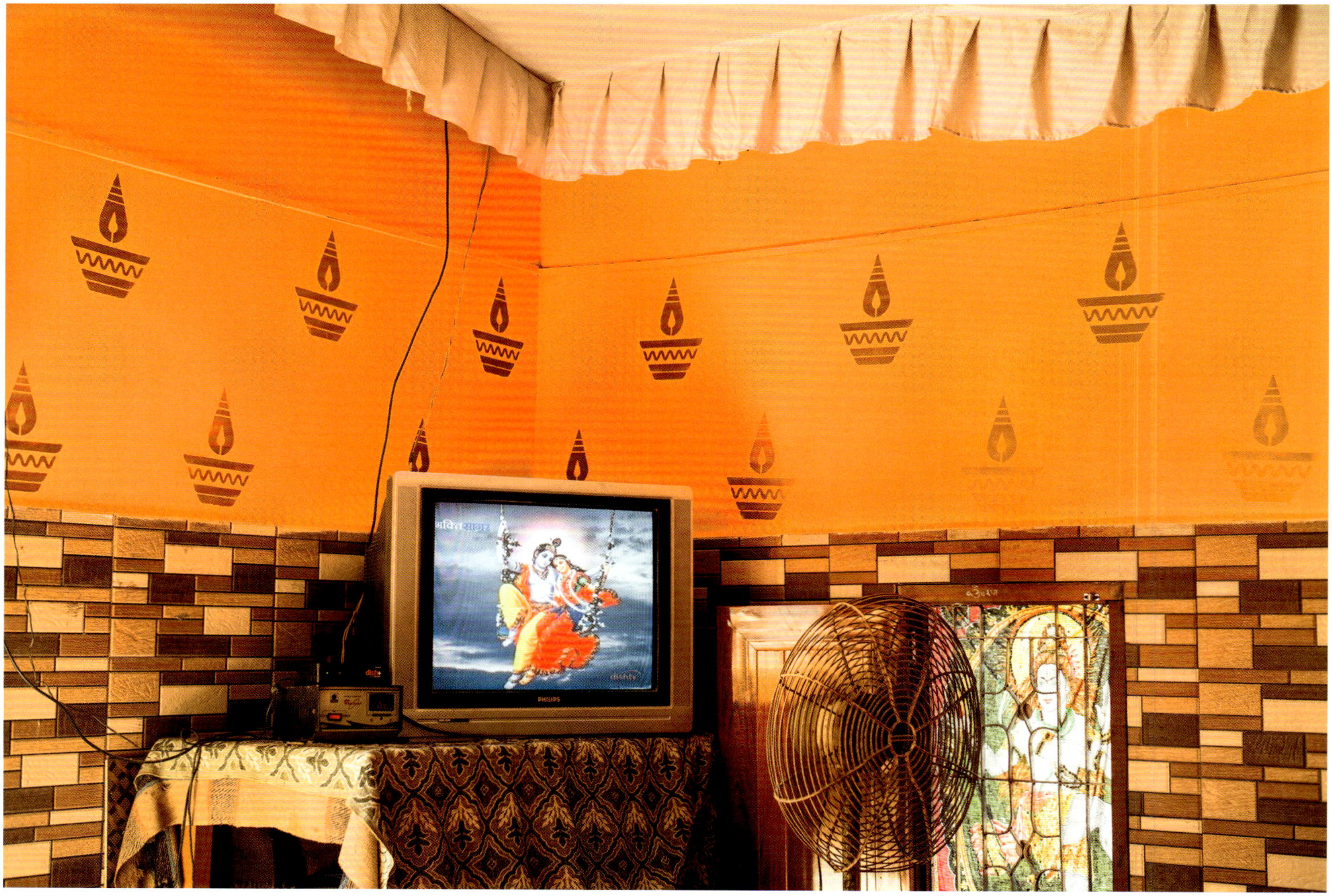
PHILIPS

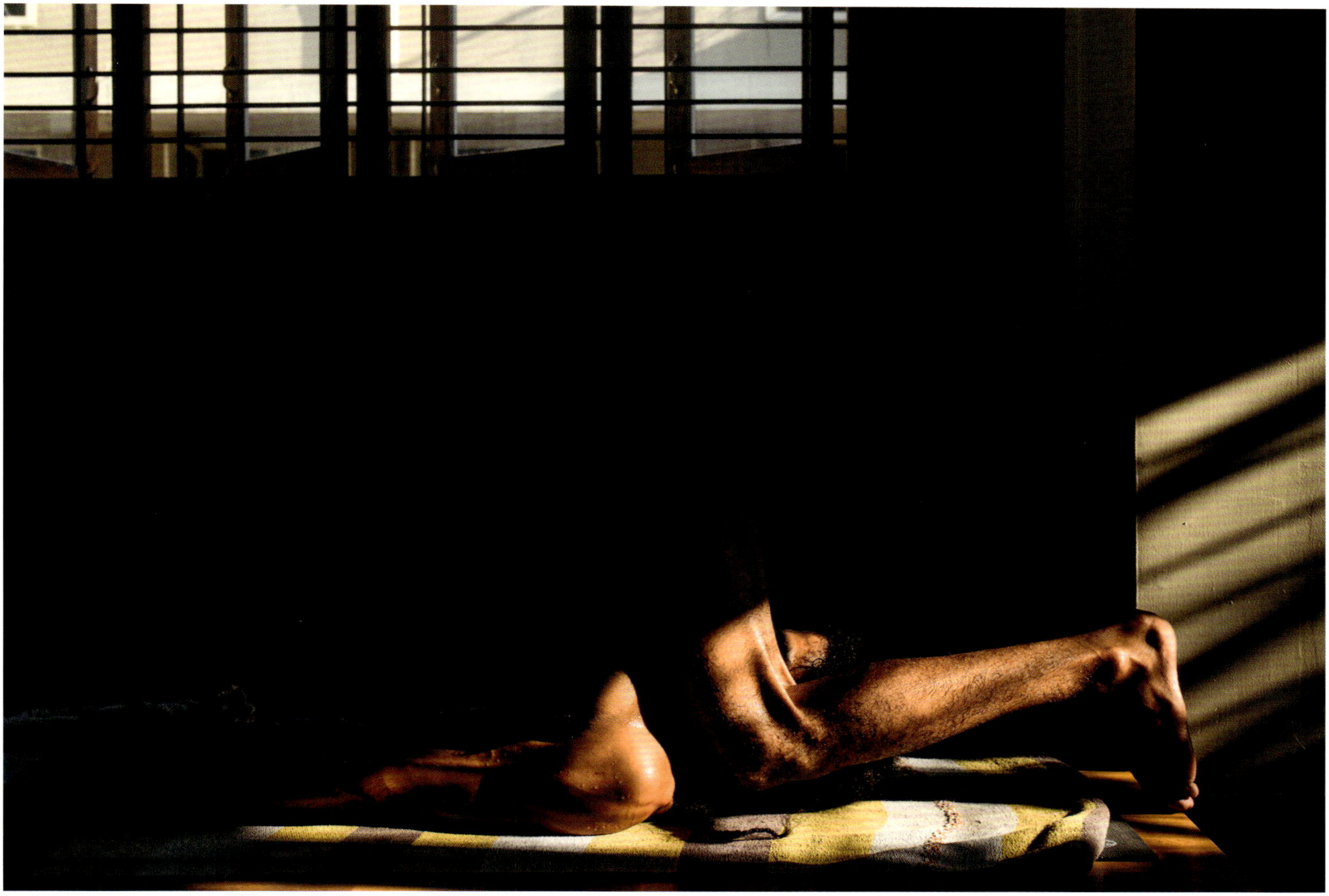

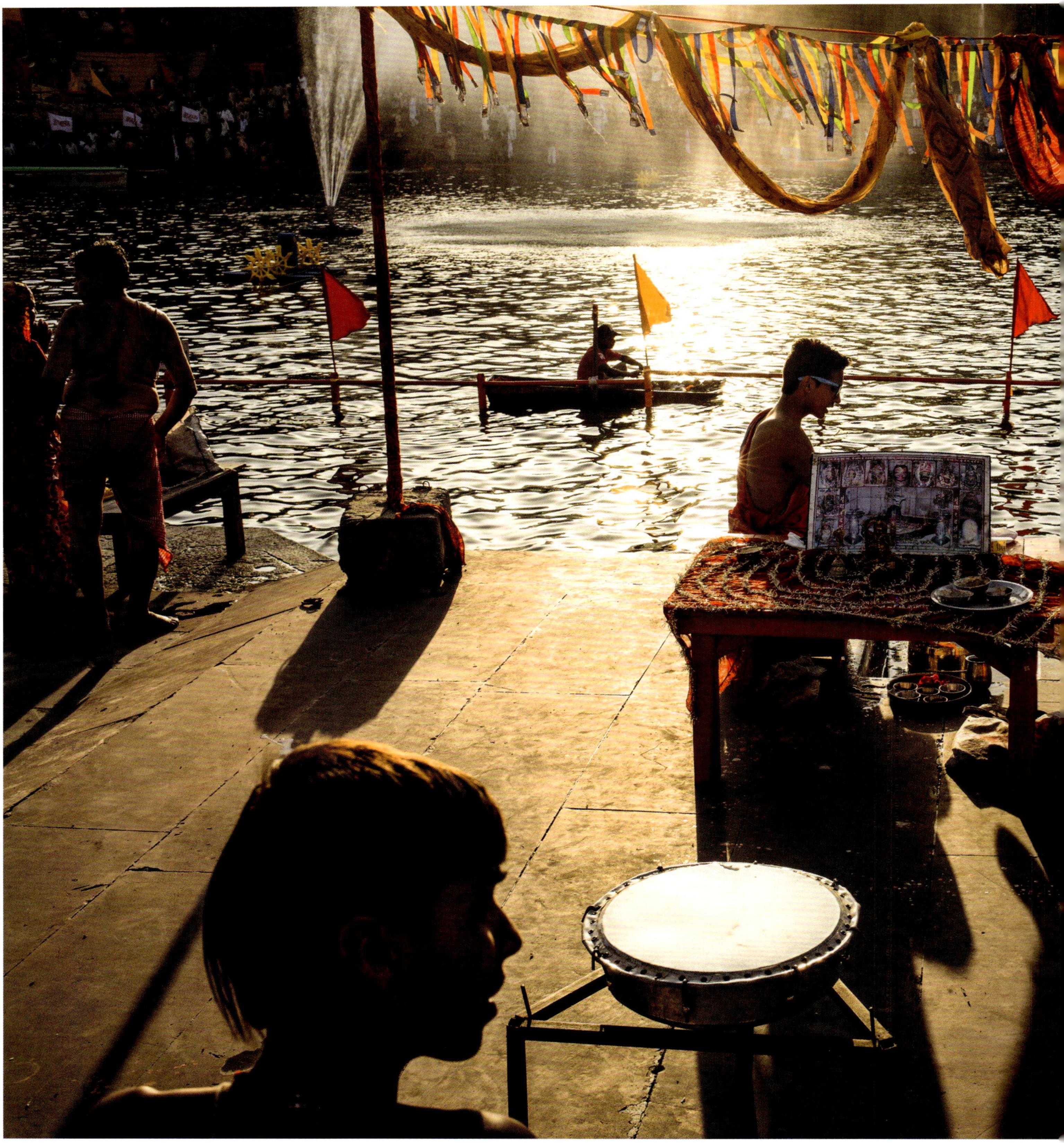

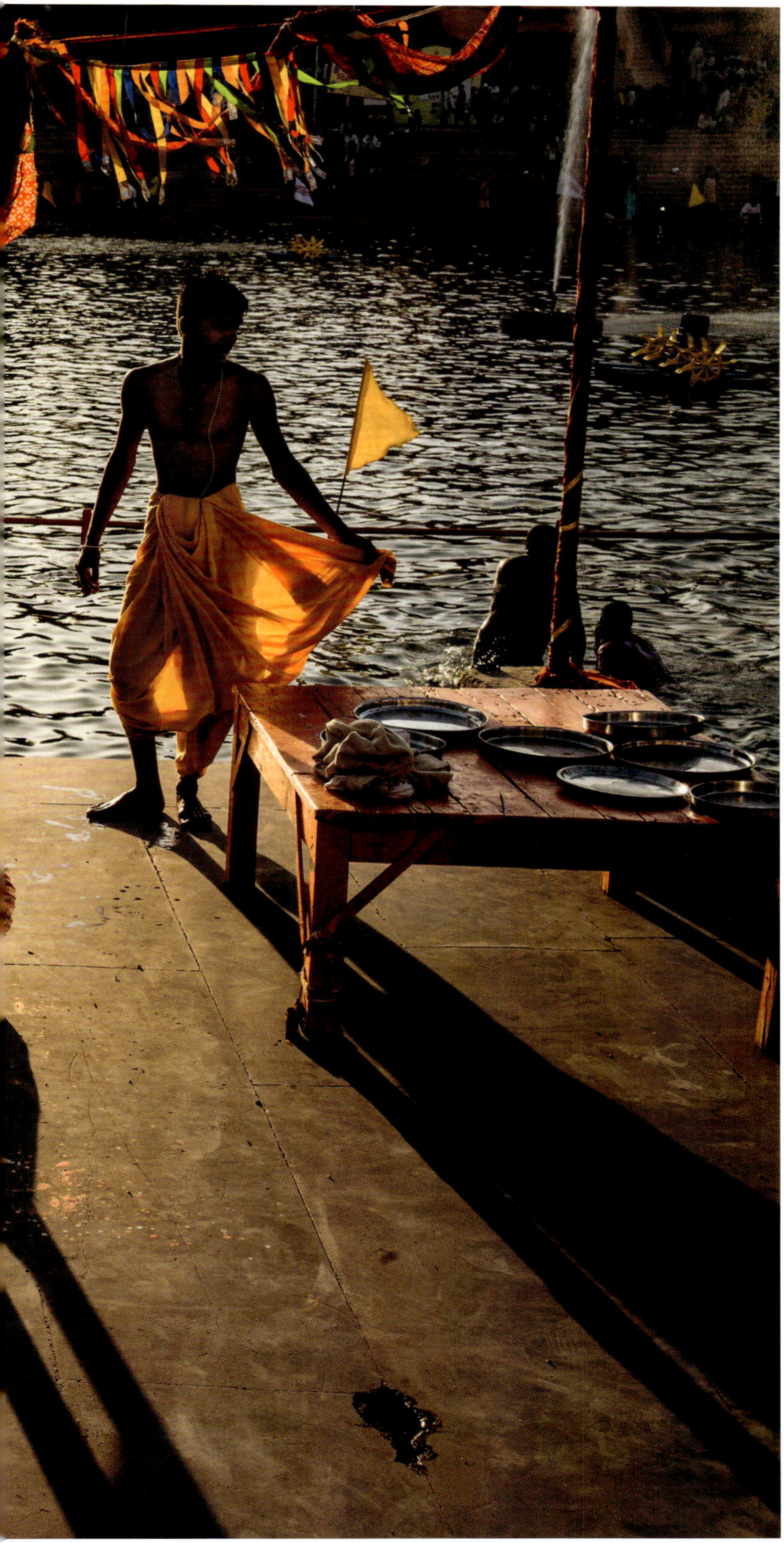

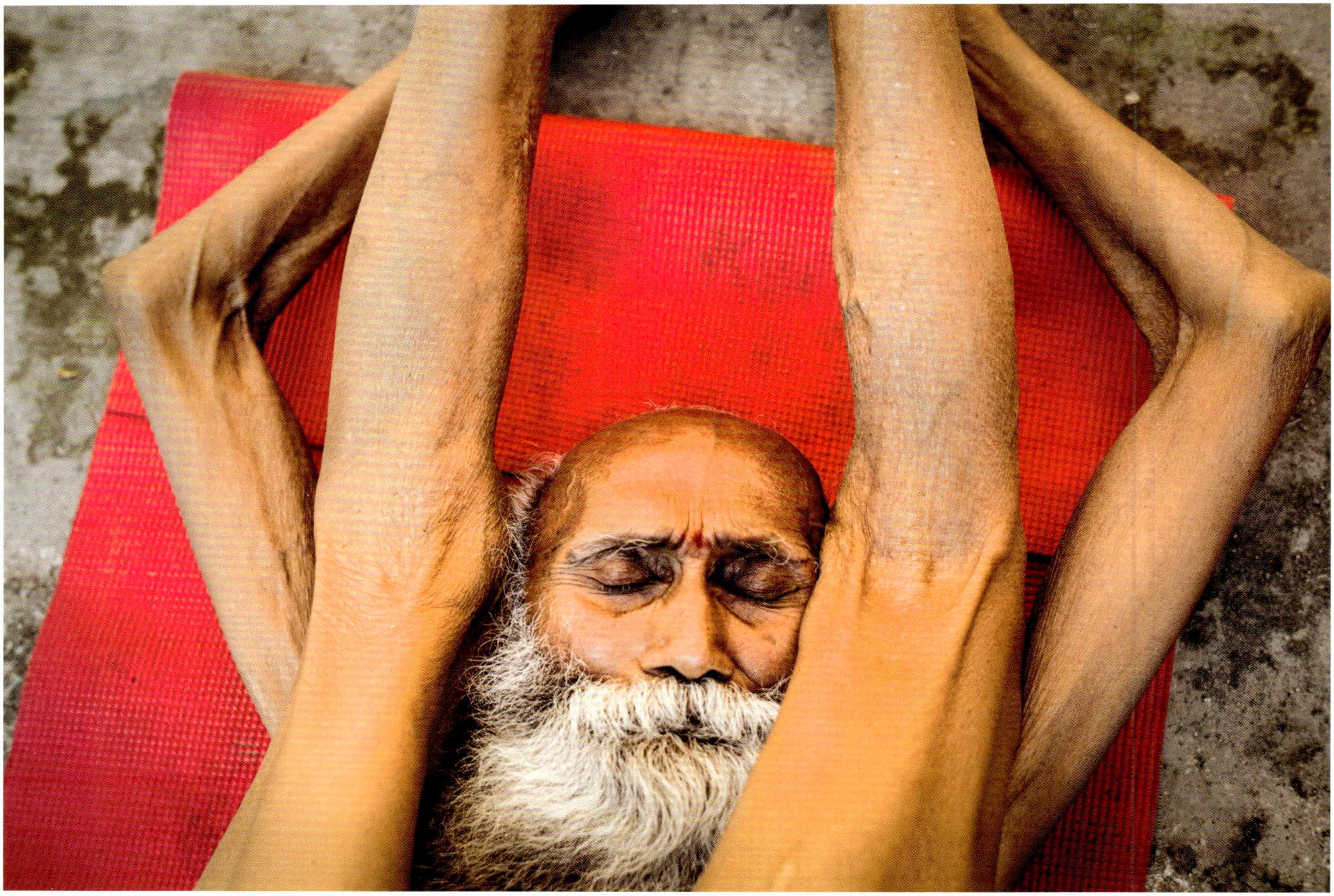

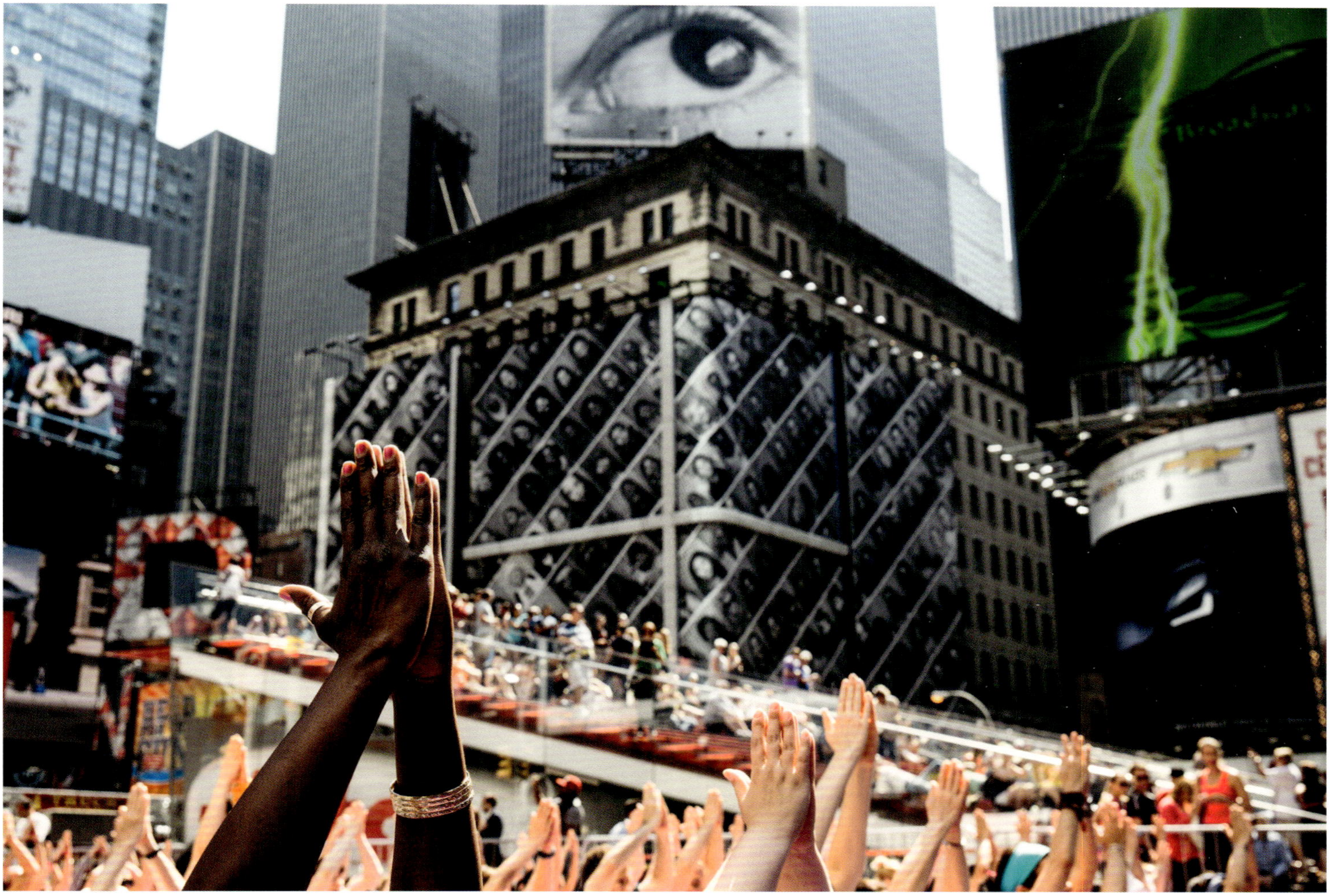

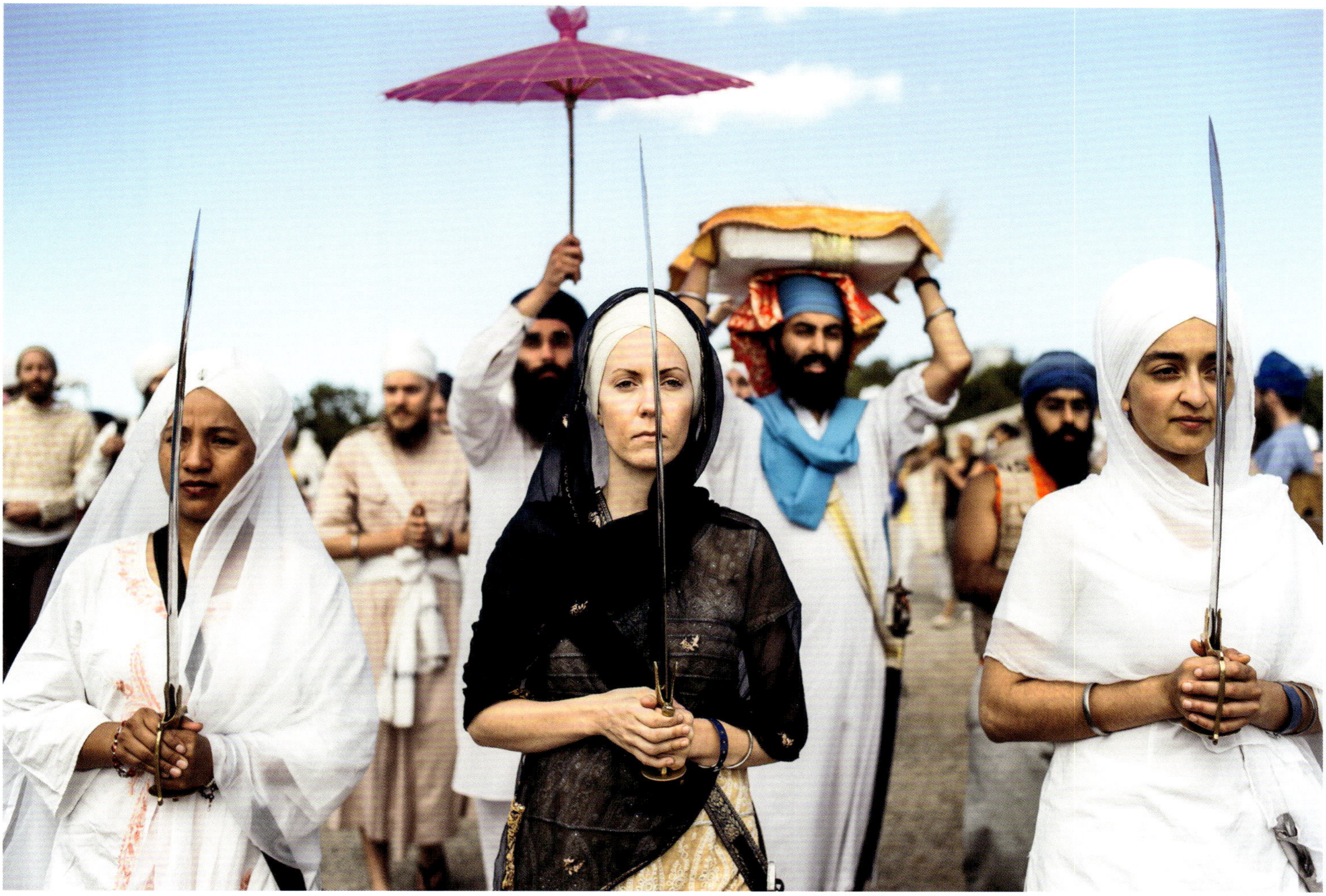

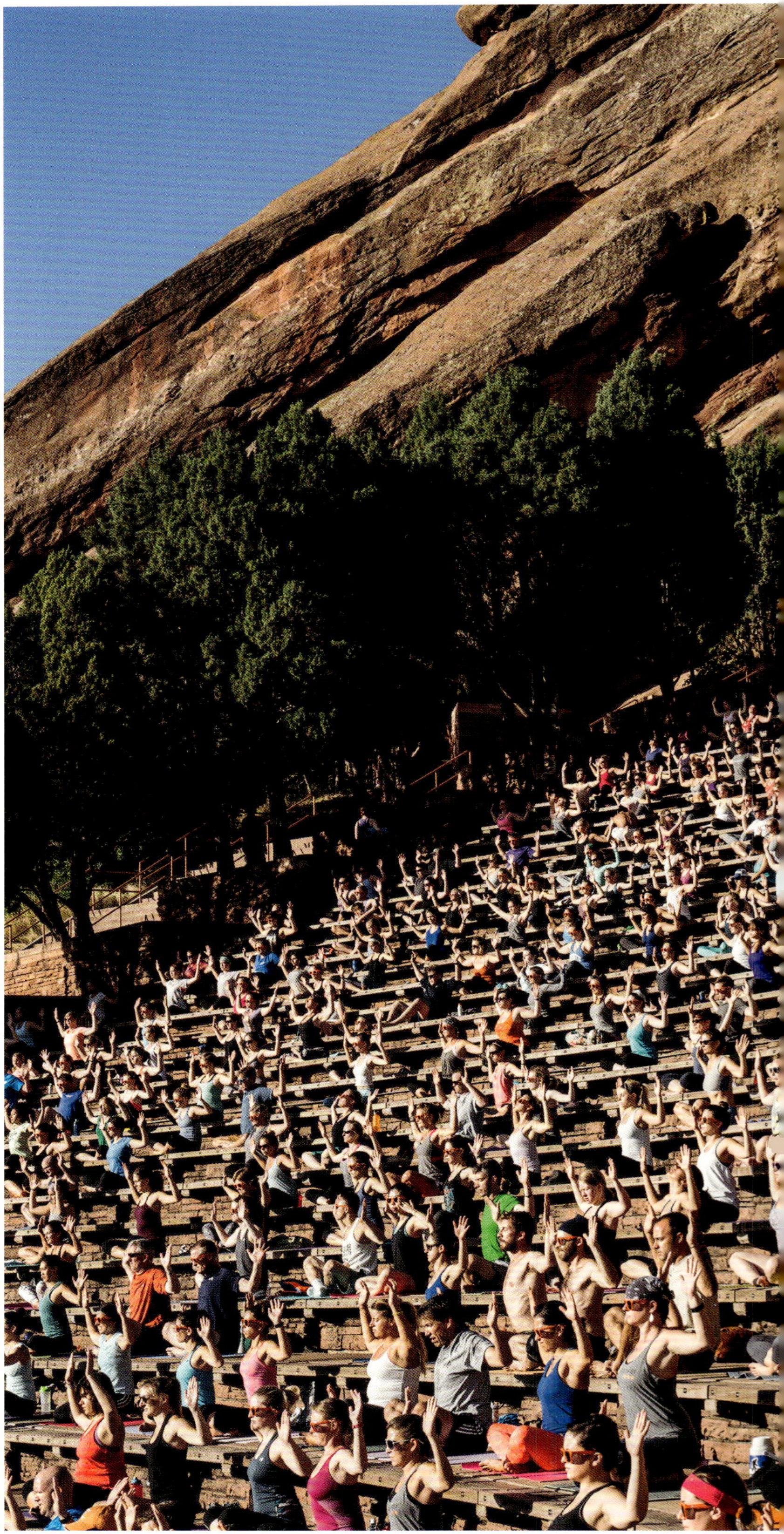

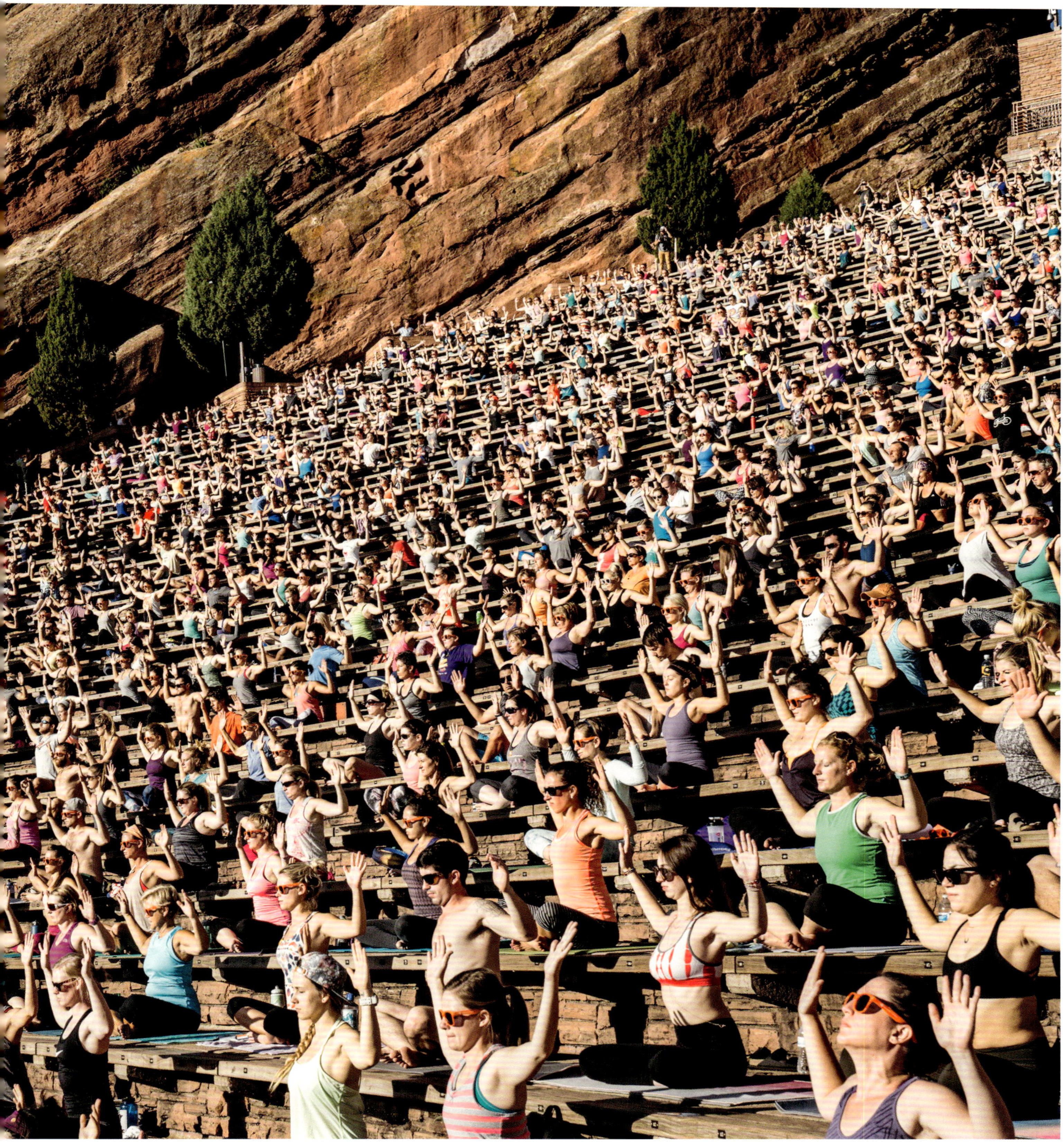

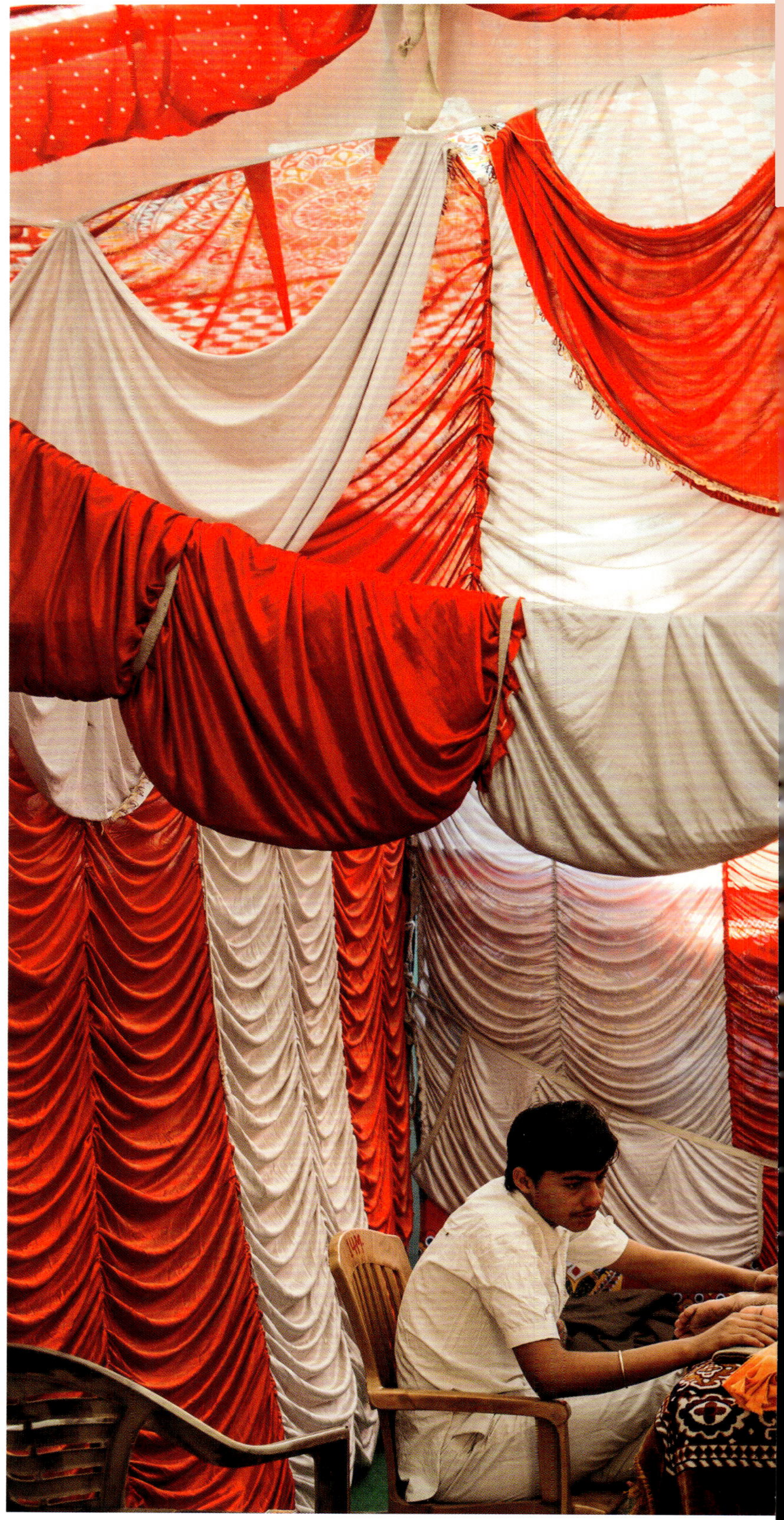

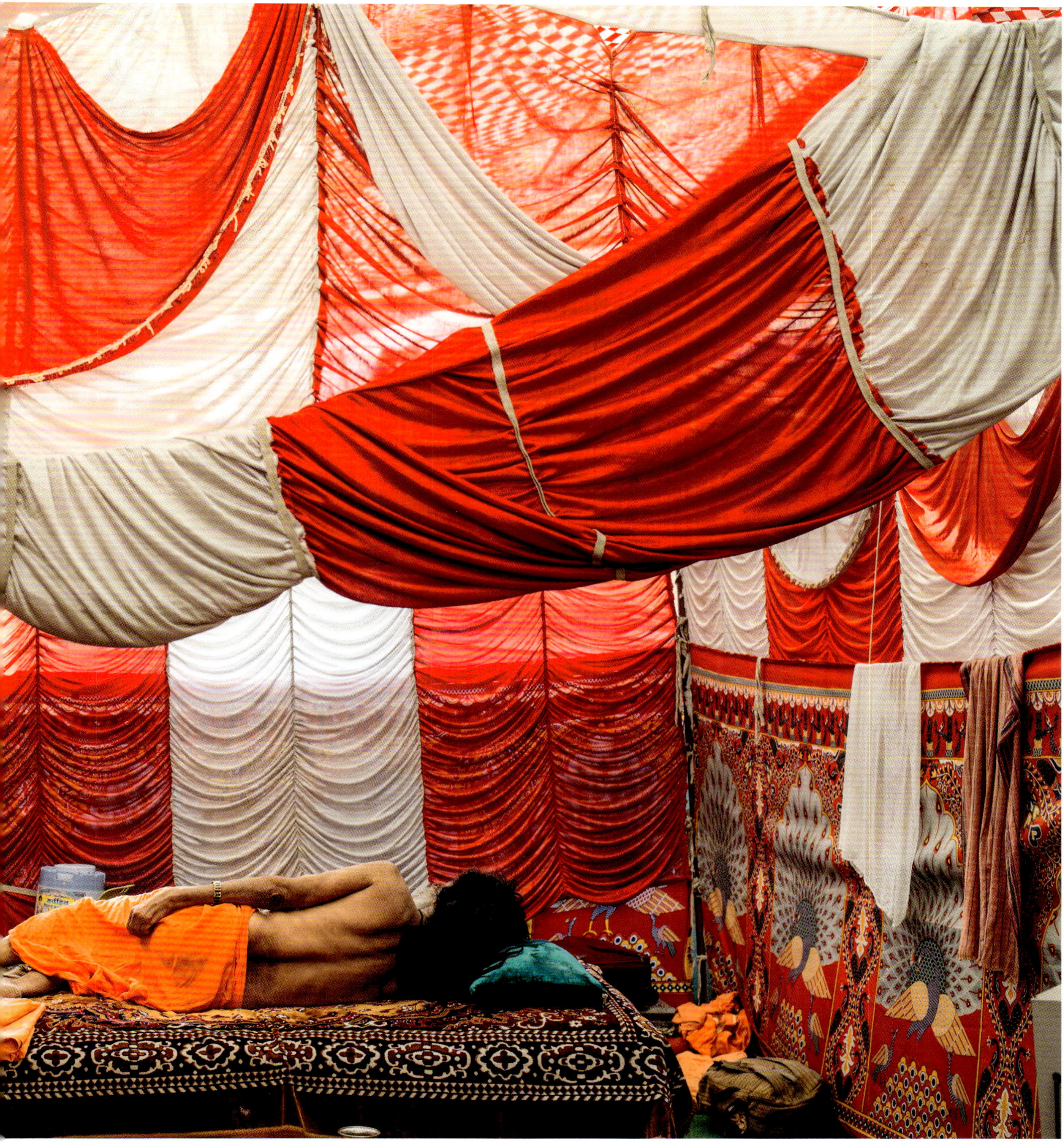

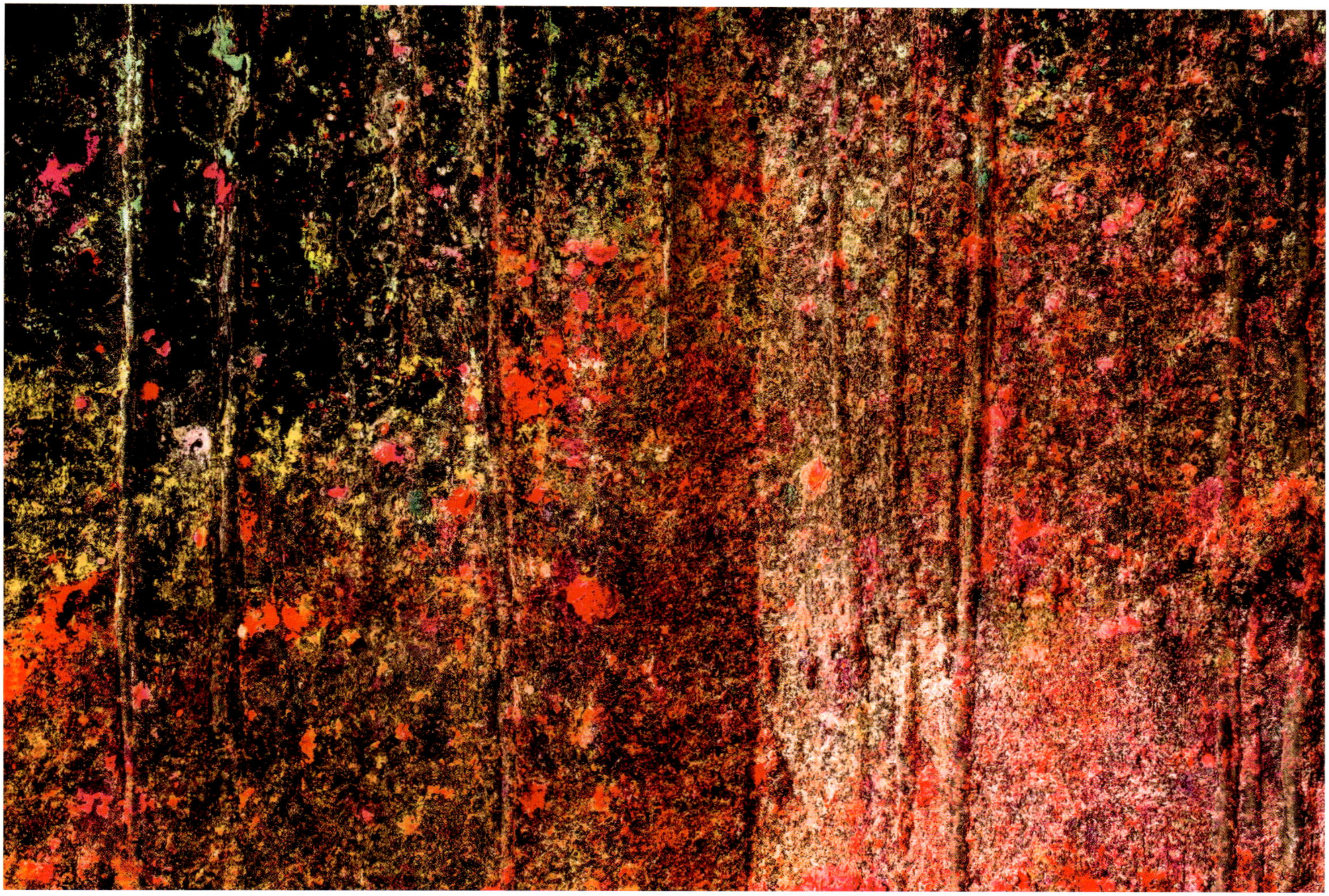

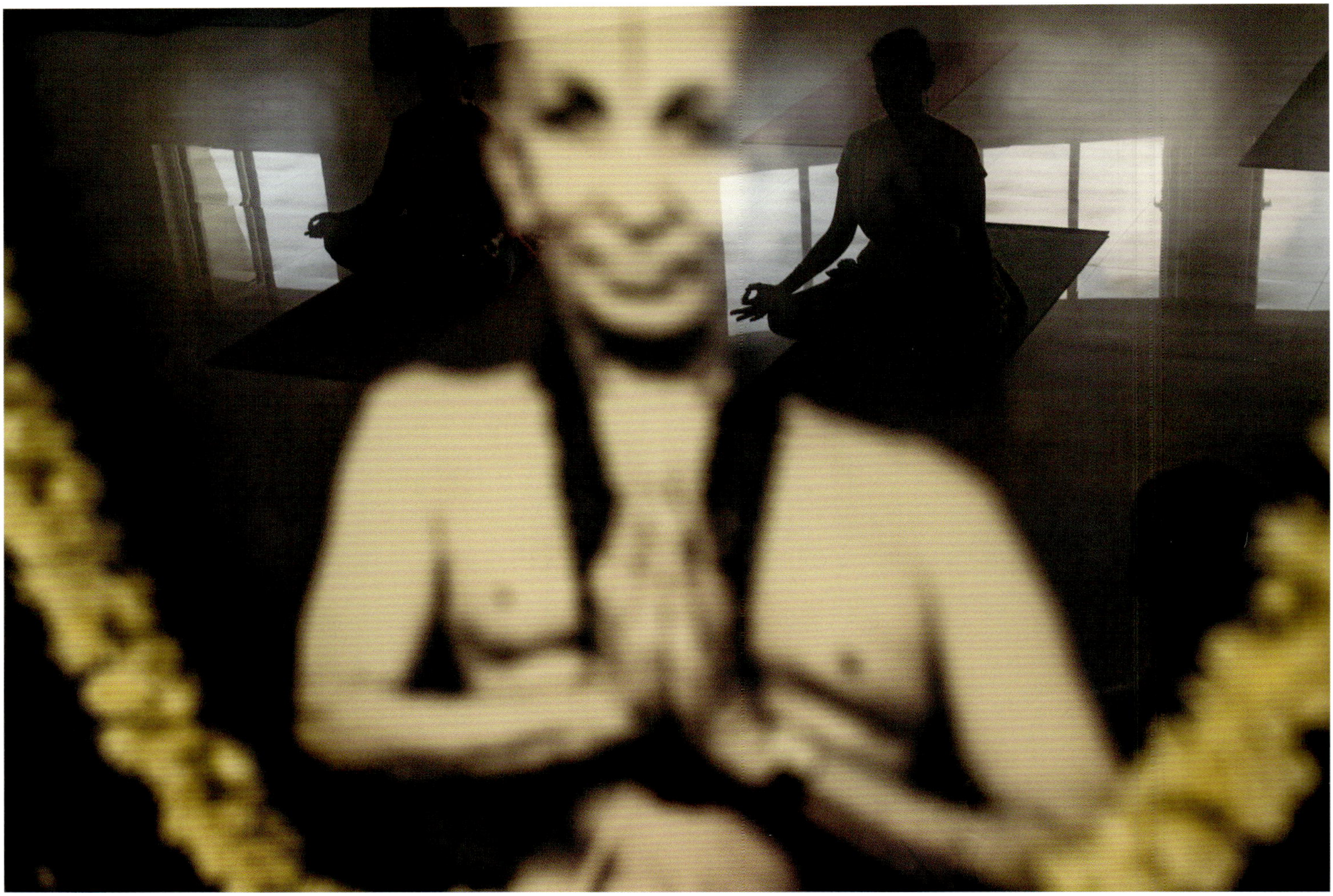

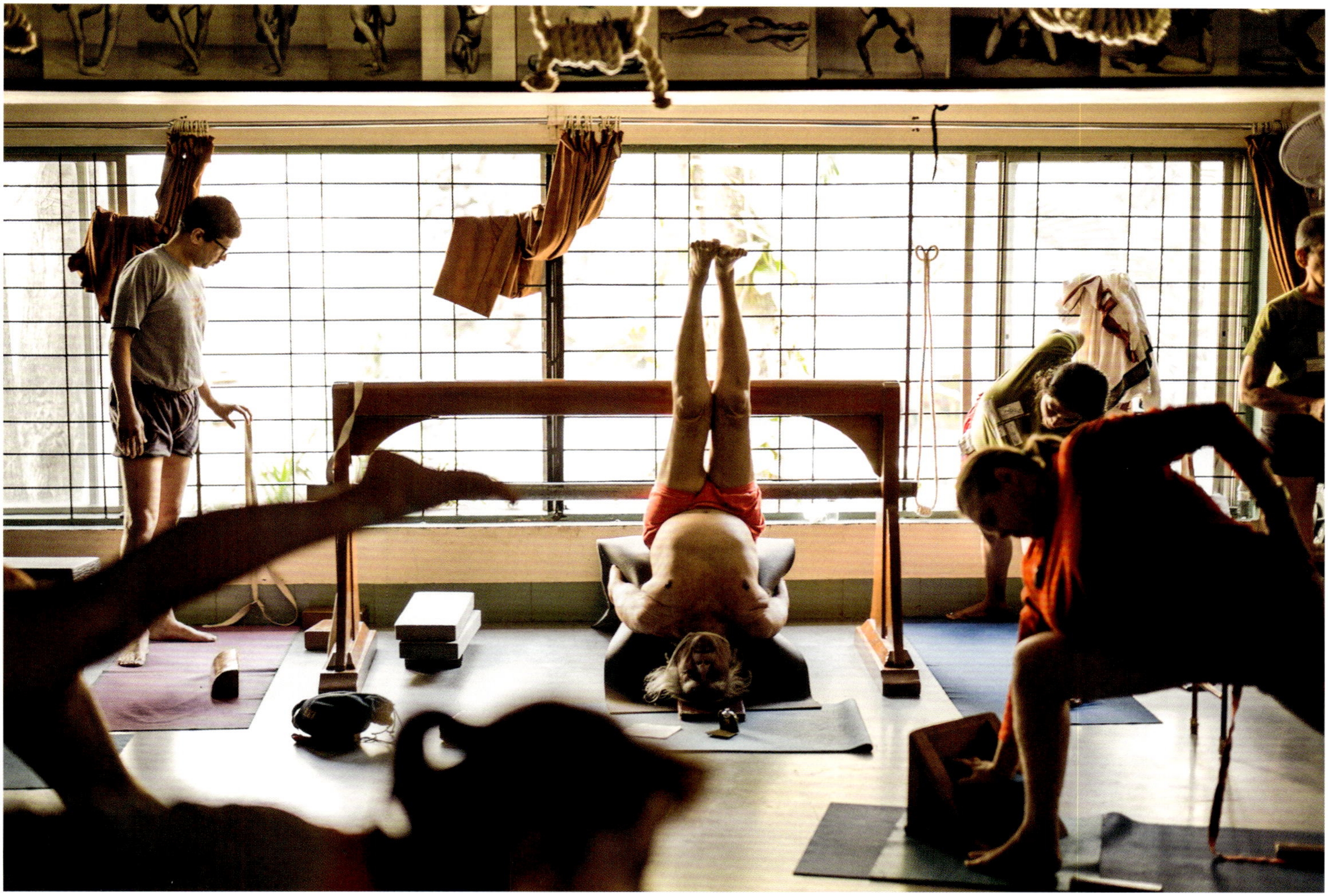

Silence is not silent.
Silence speaks.
It speaks most eloquently.

Silence is not still.
Silence leads.
It leads most perfectly.

Sri Chinmoy

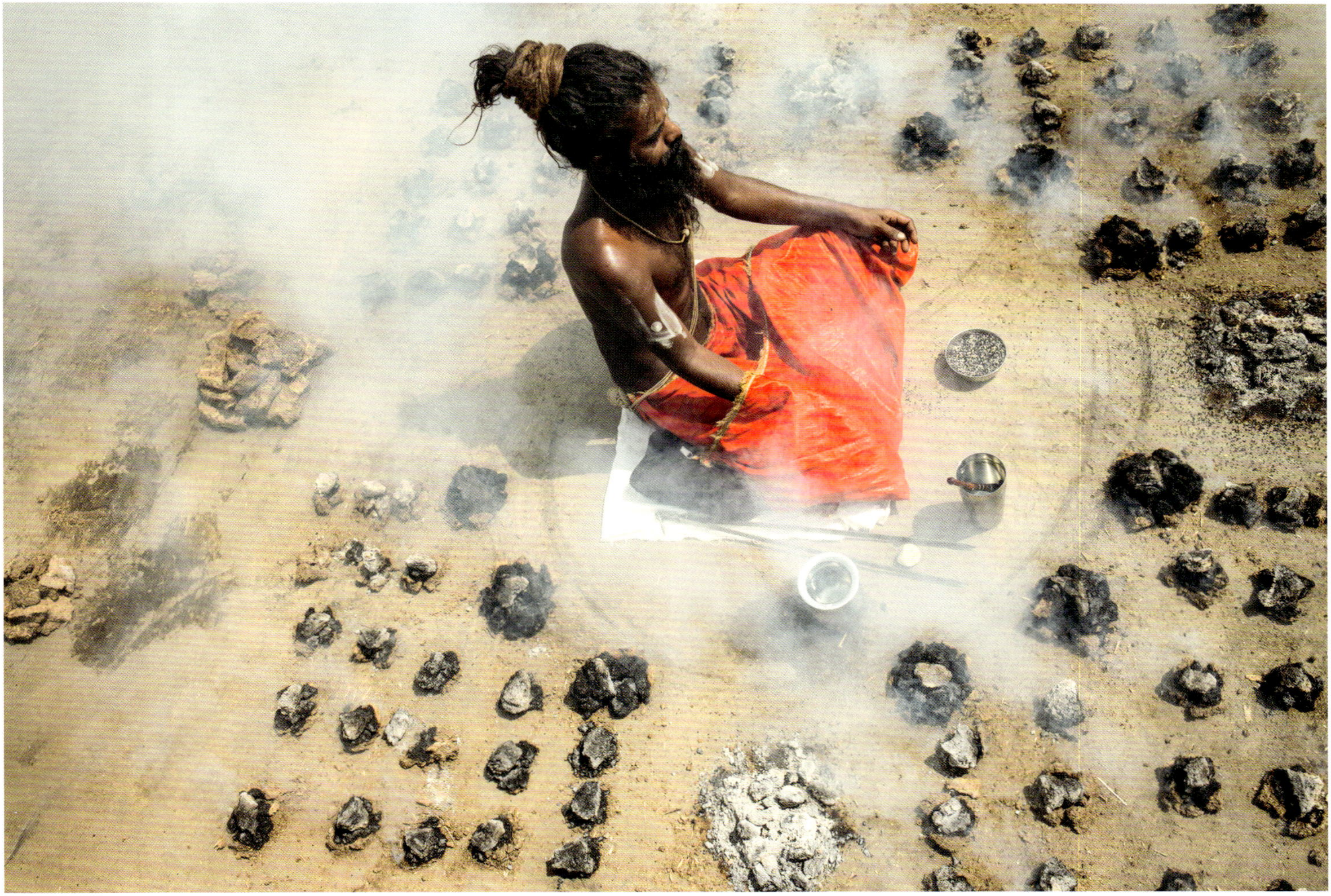

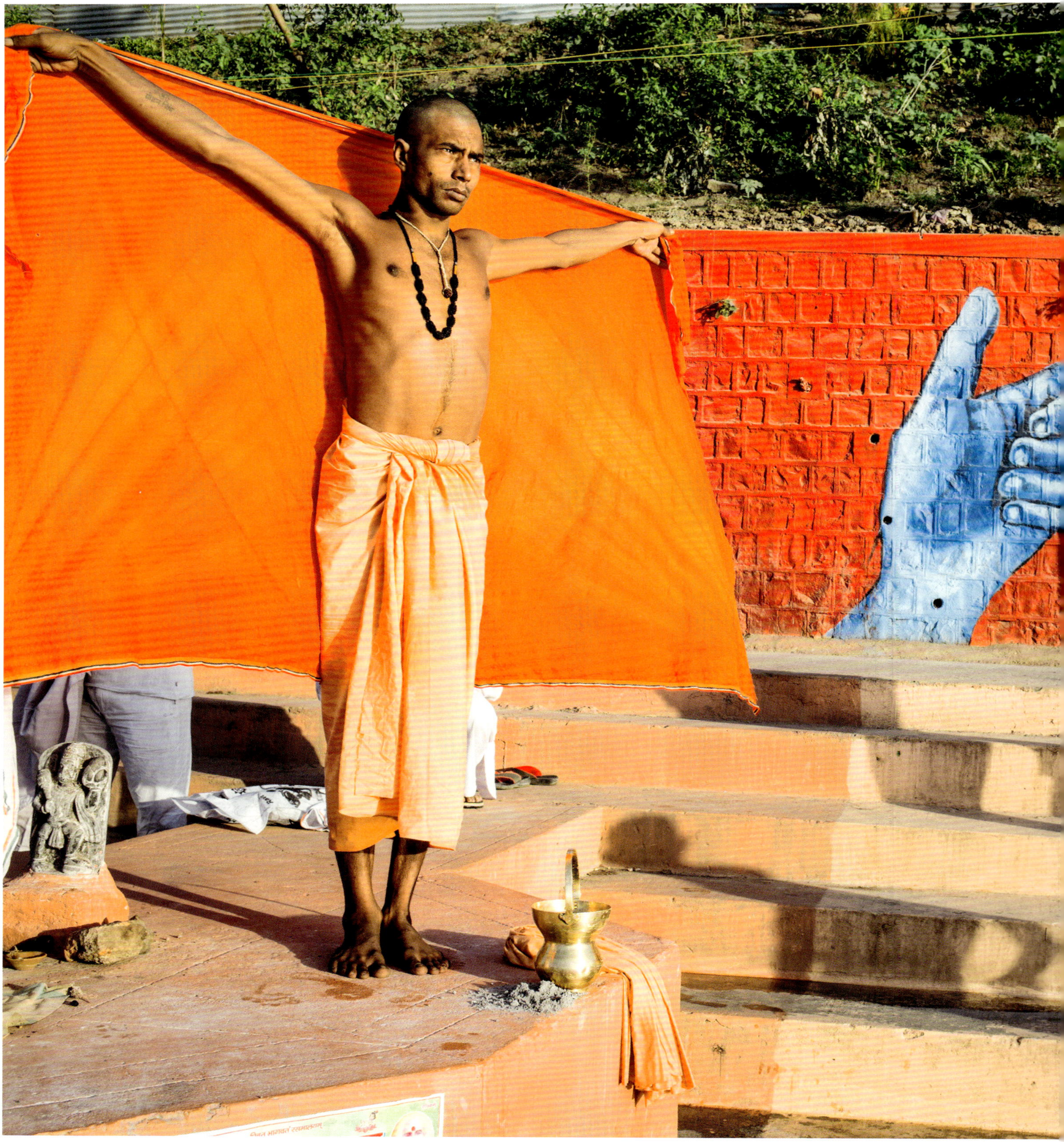

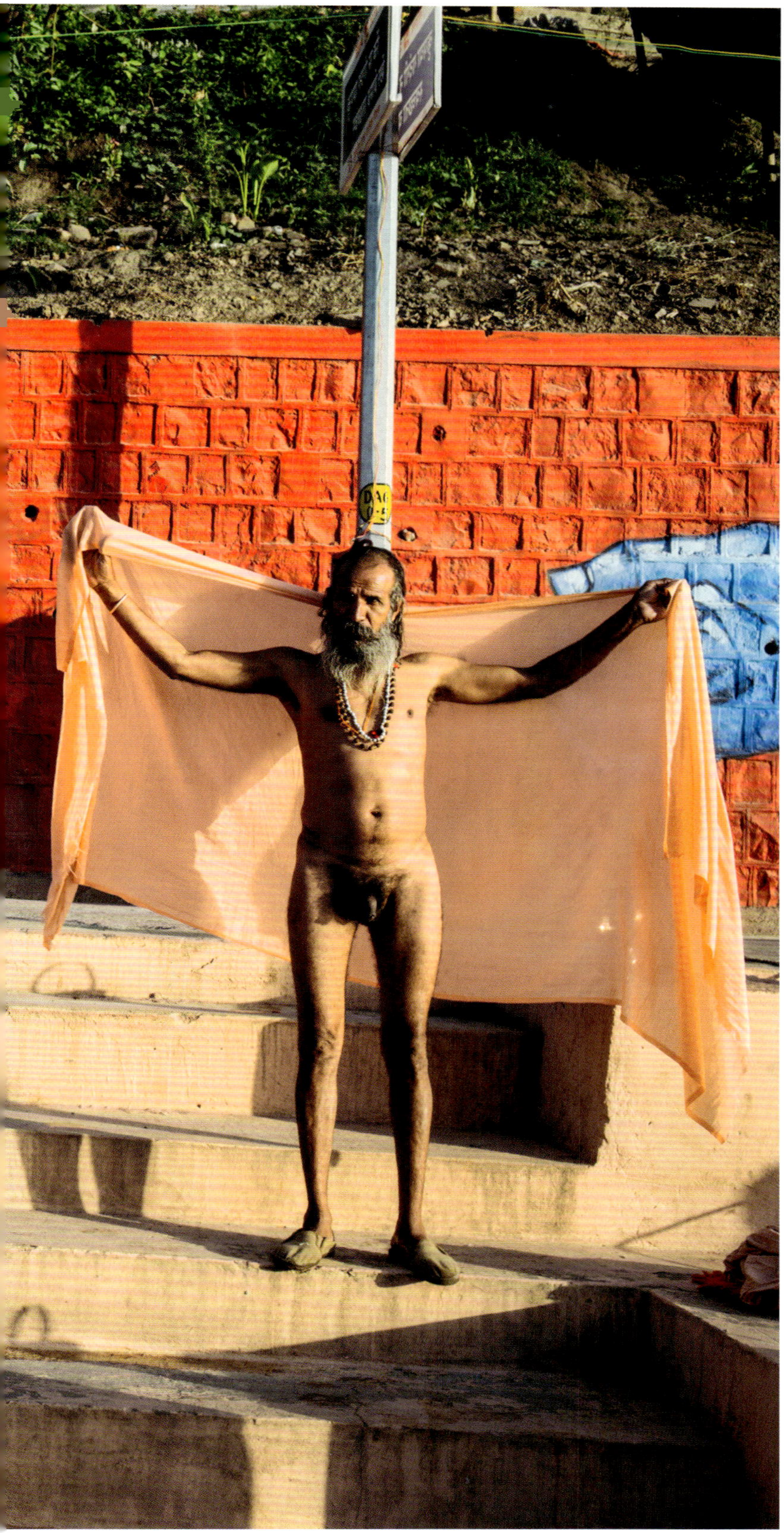

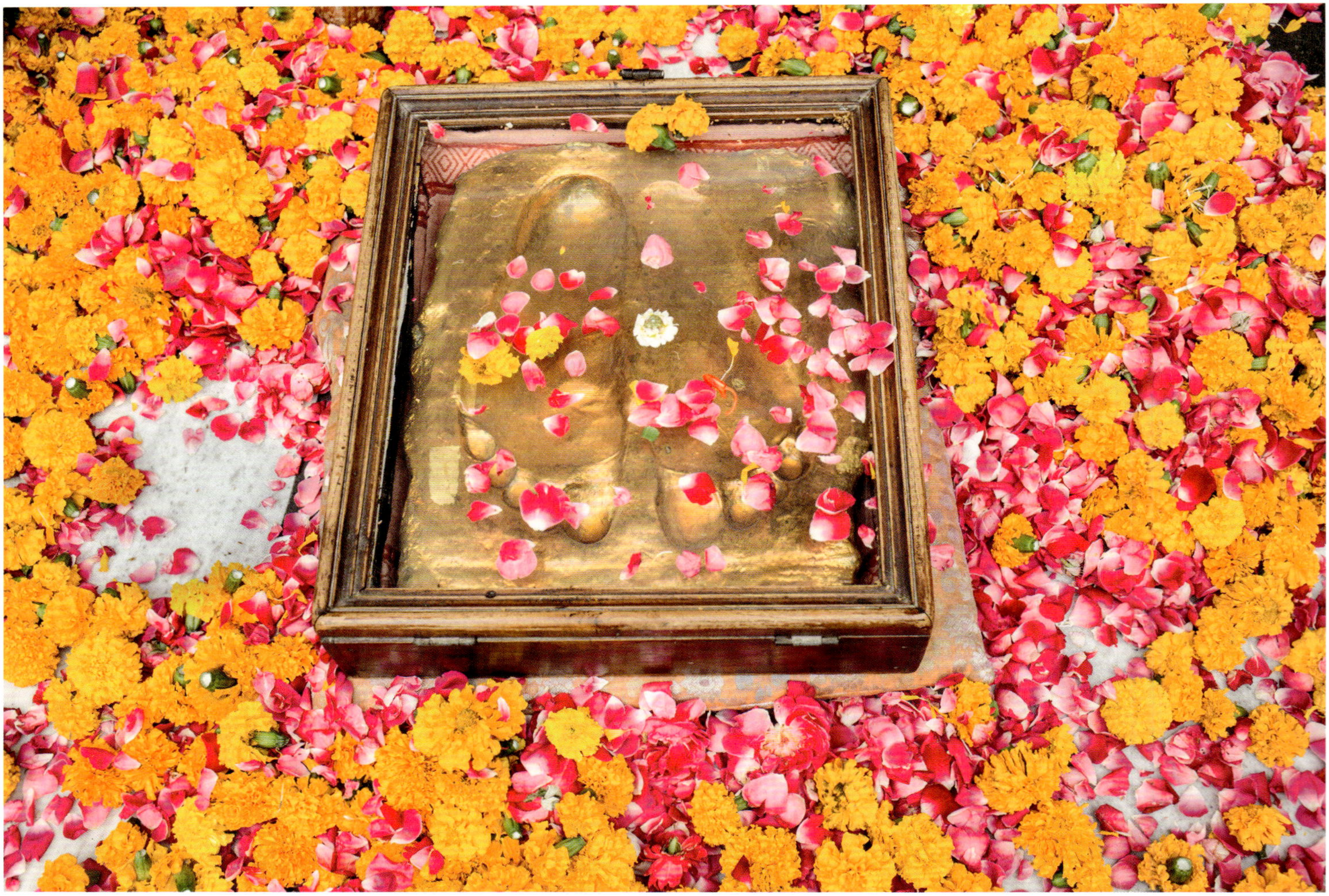

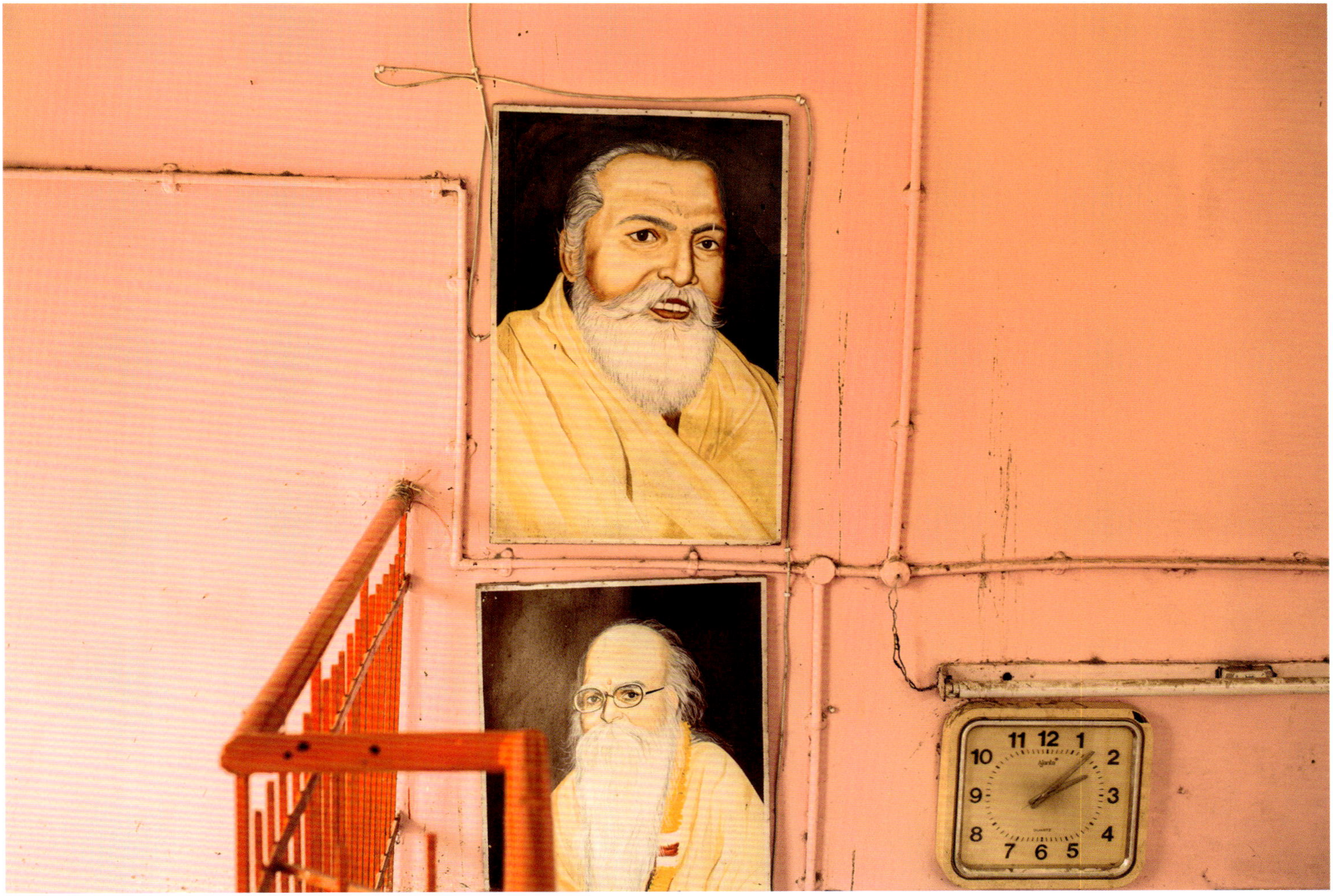

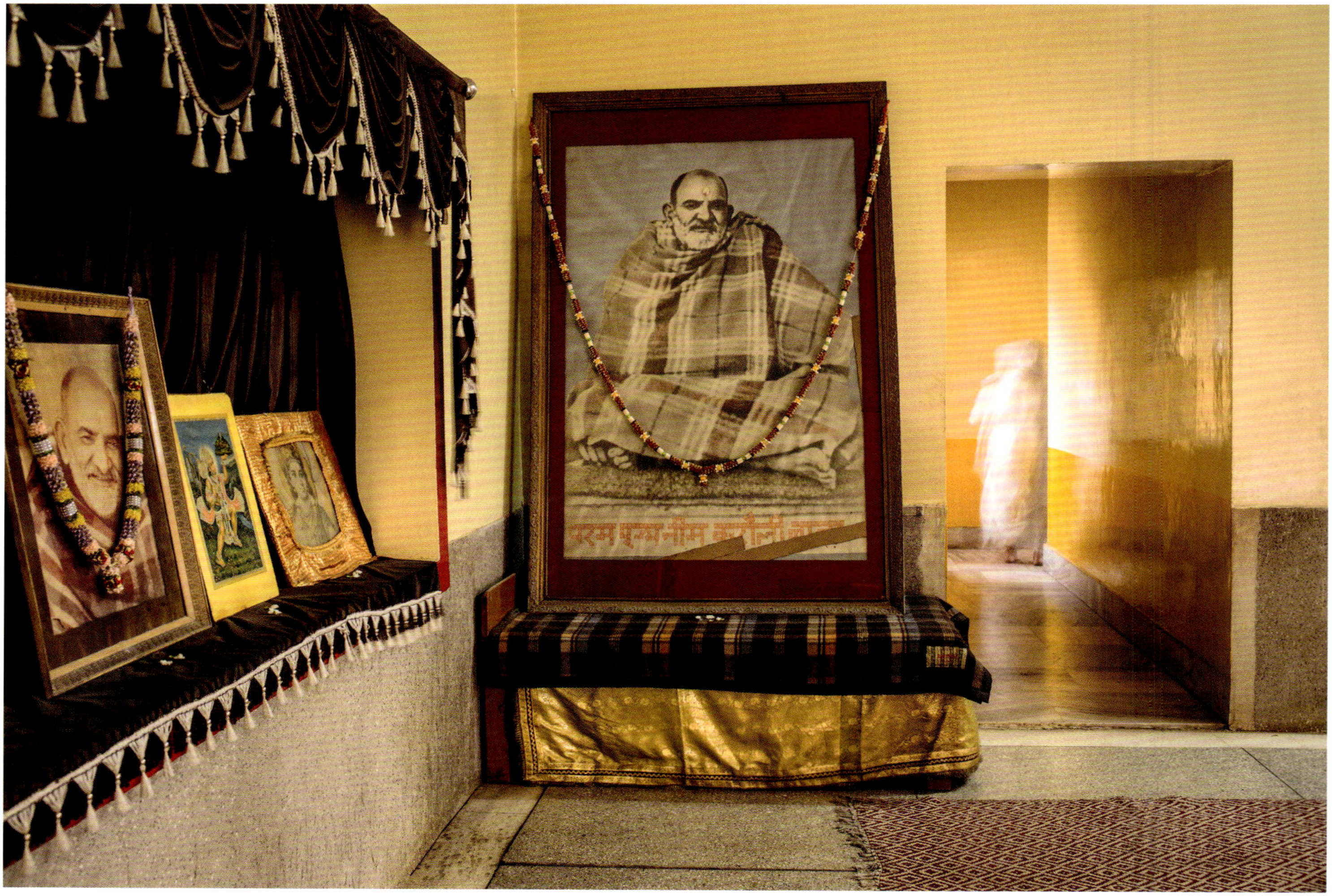
परम पूज्य नीम

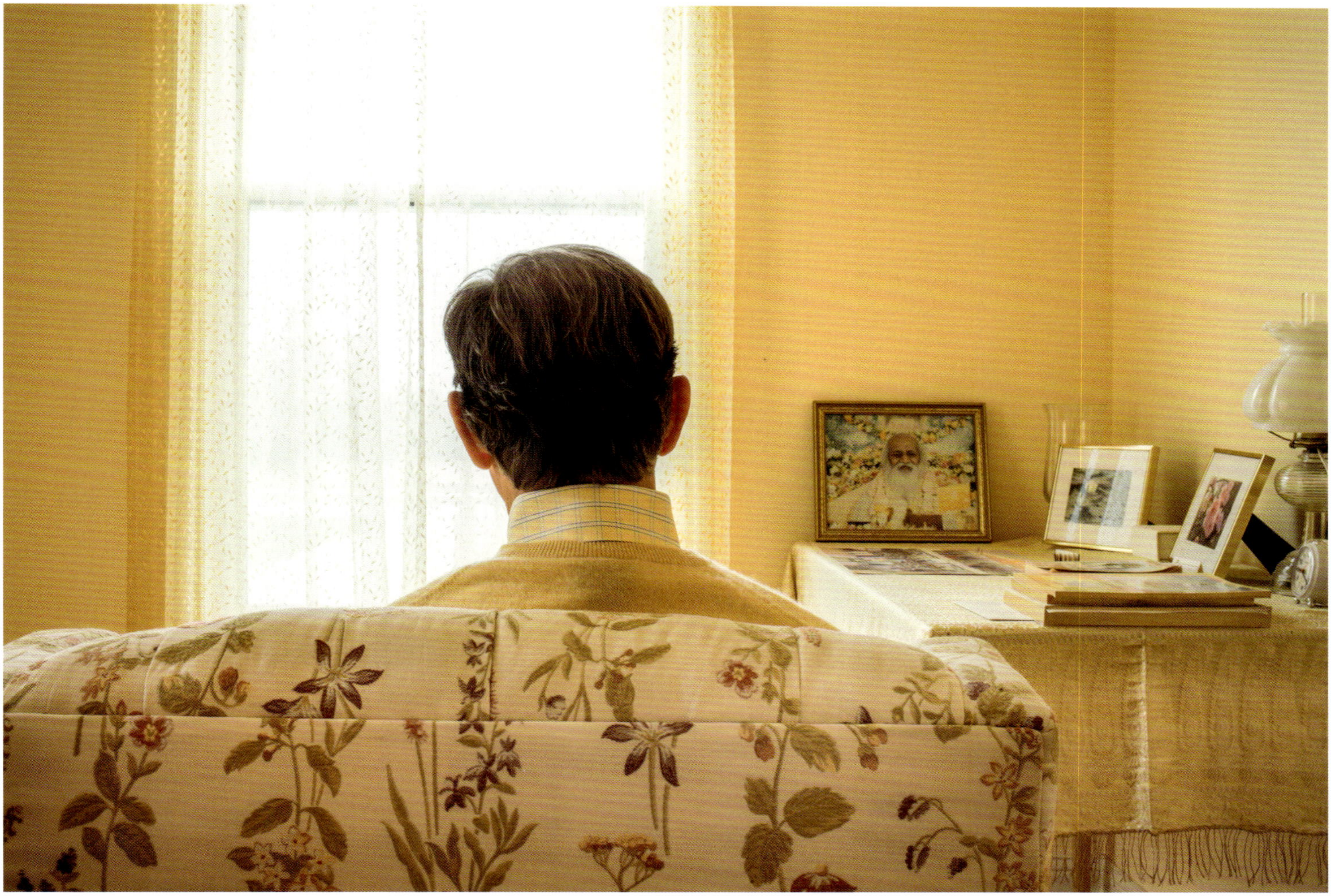

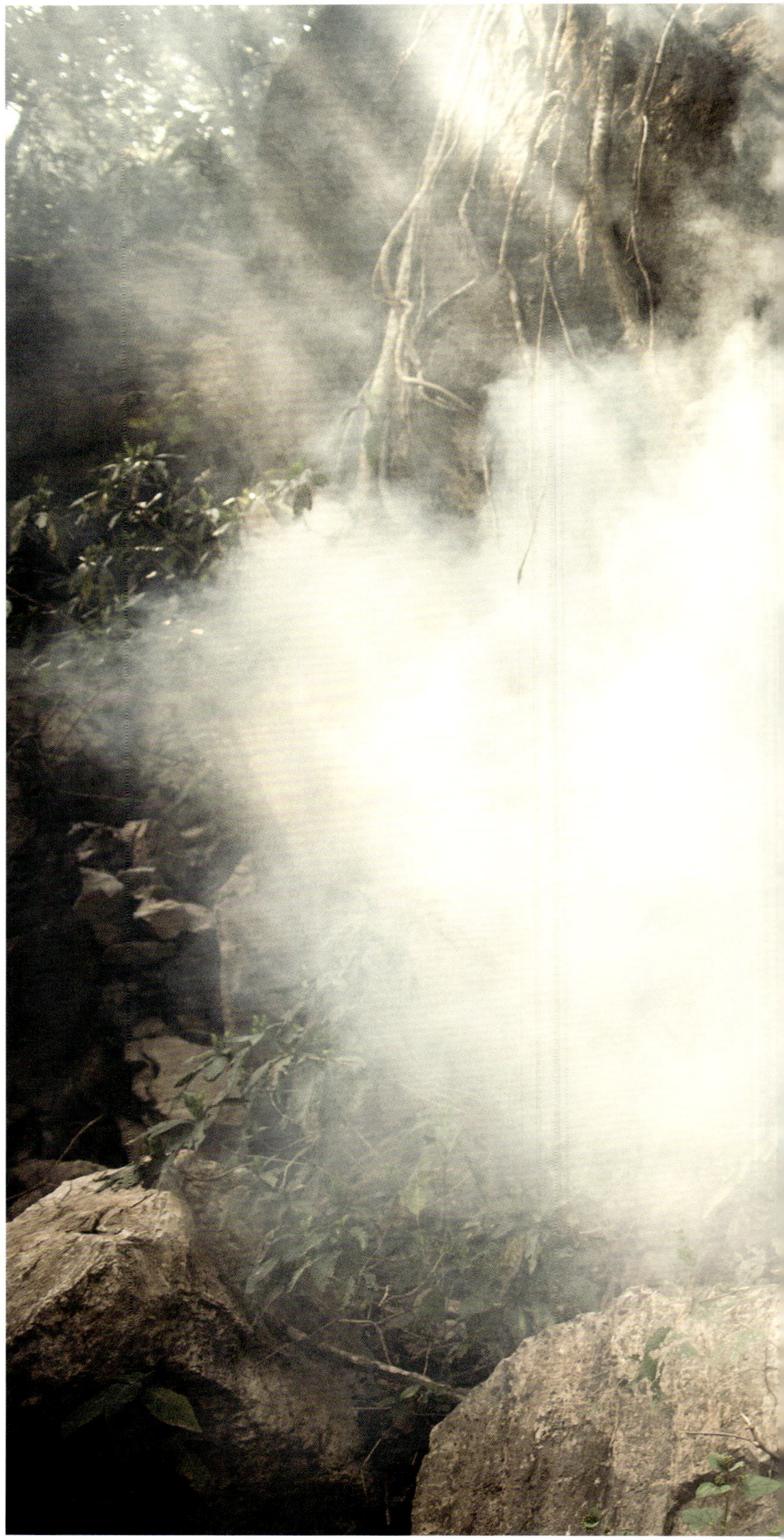

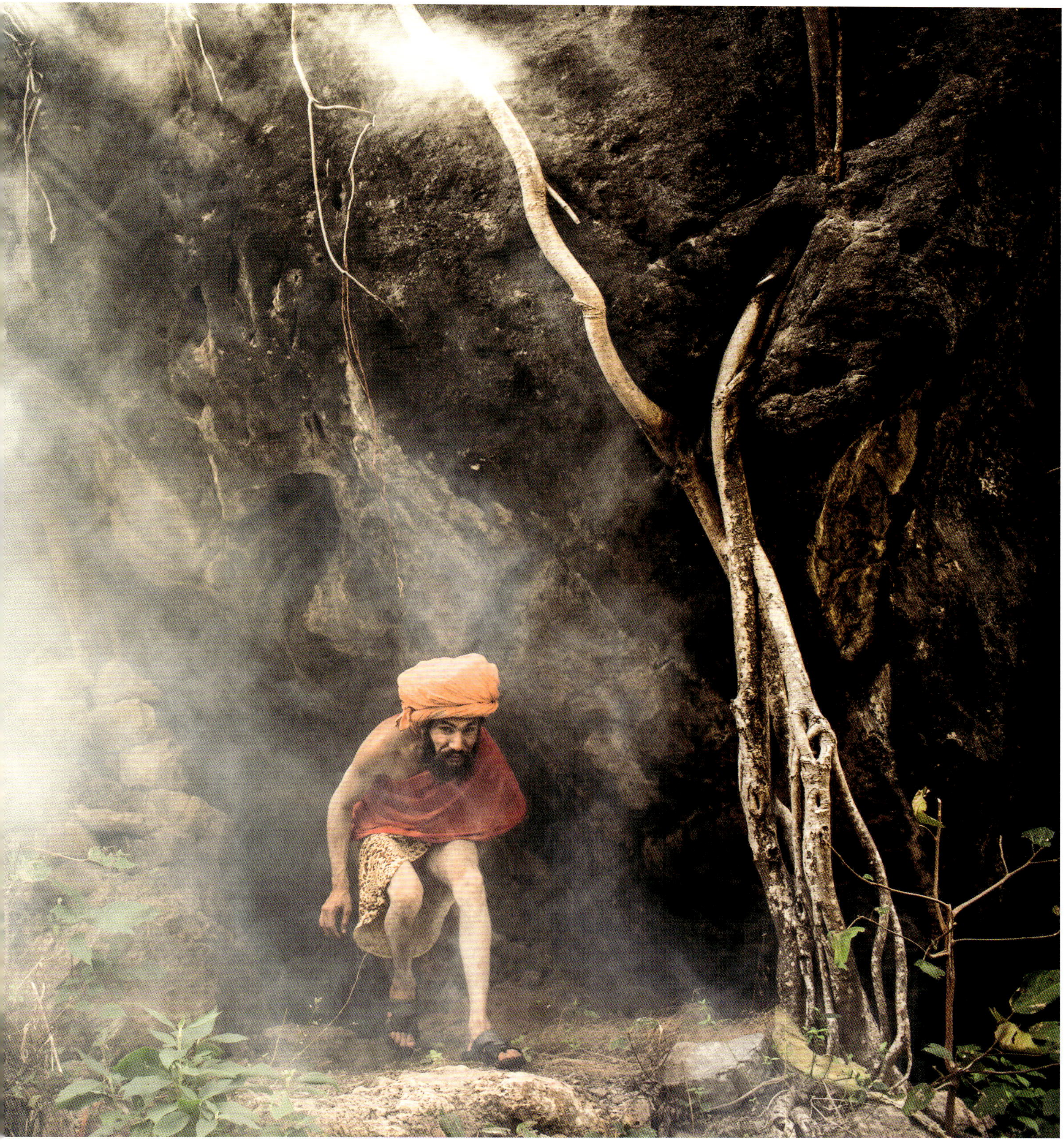

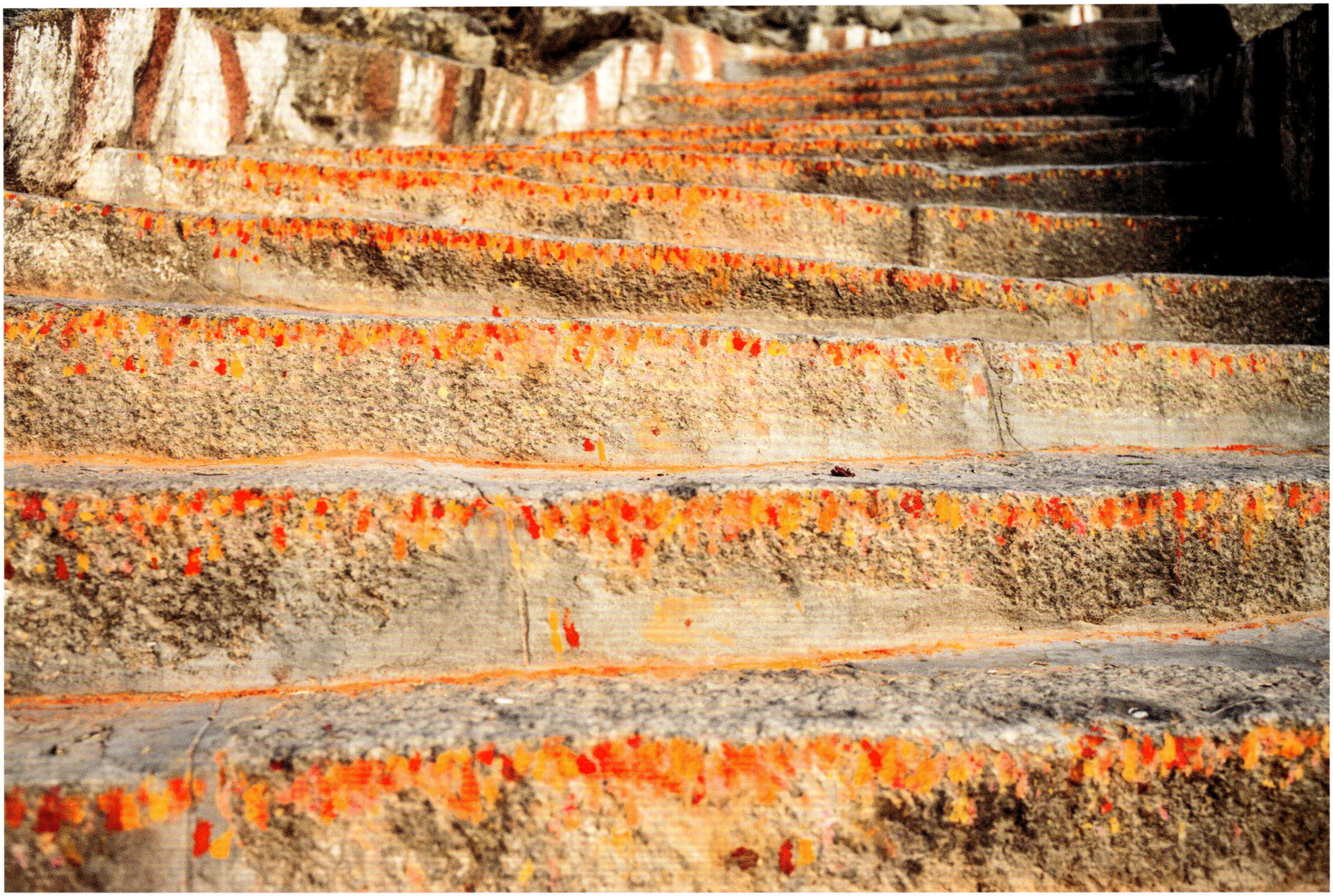

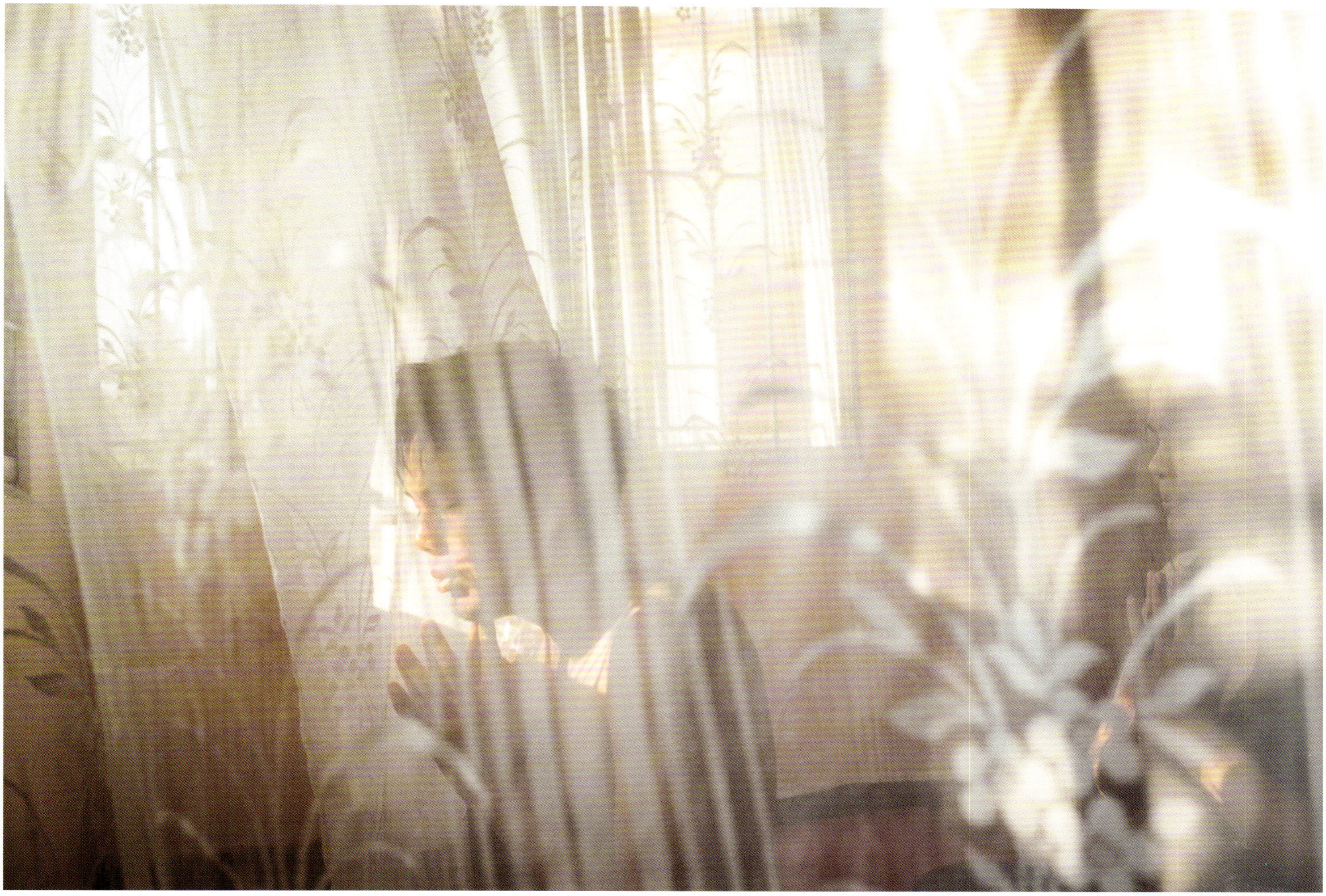

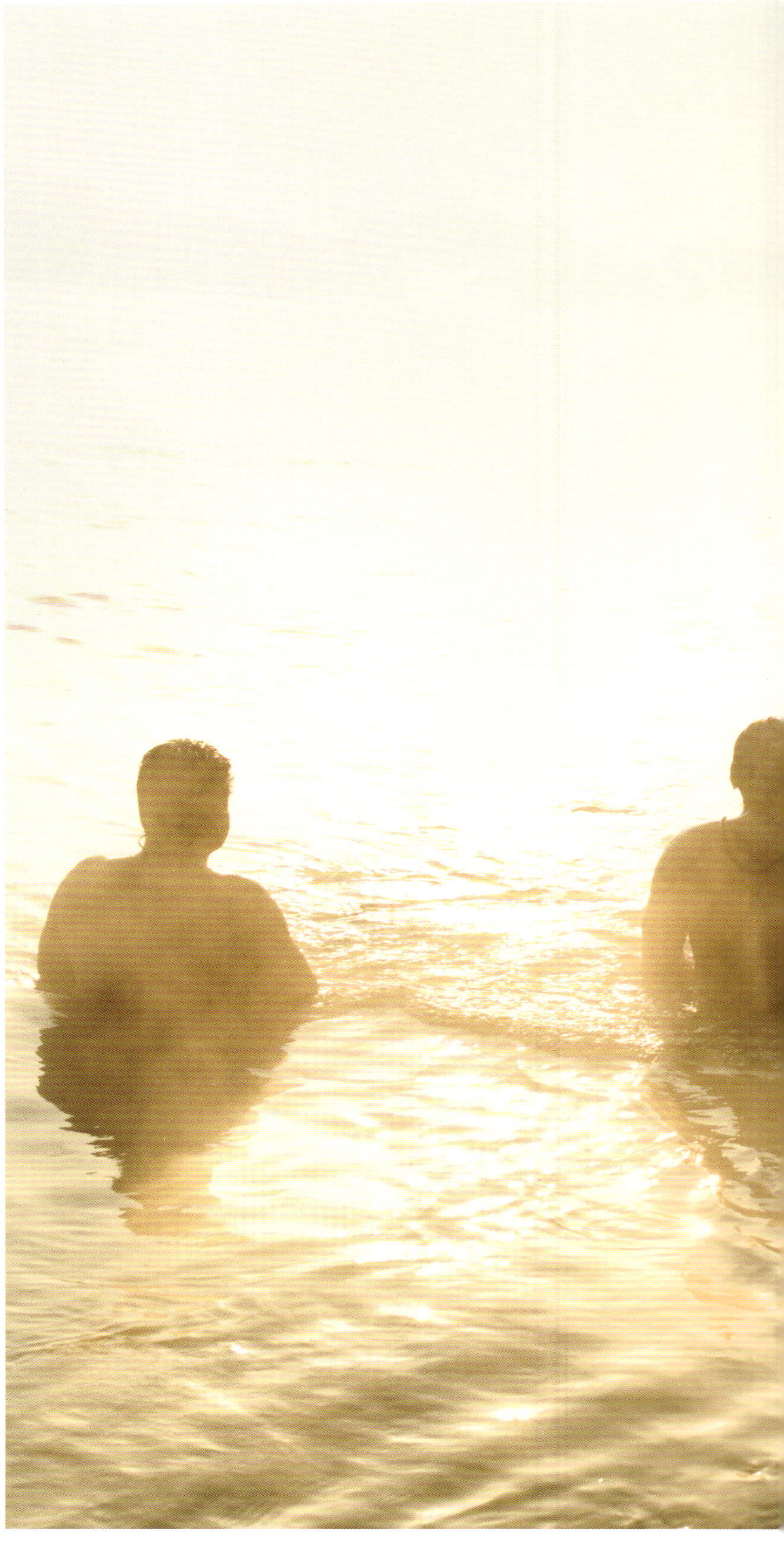

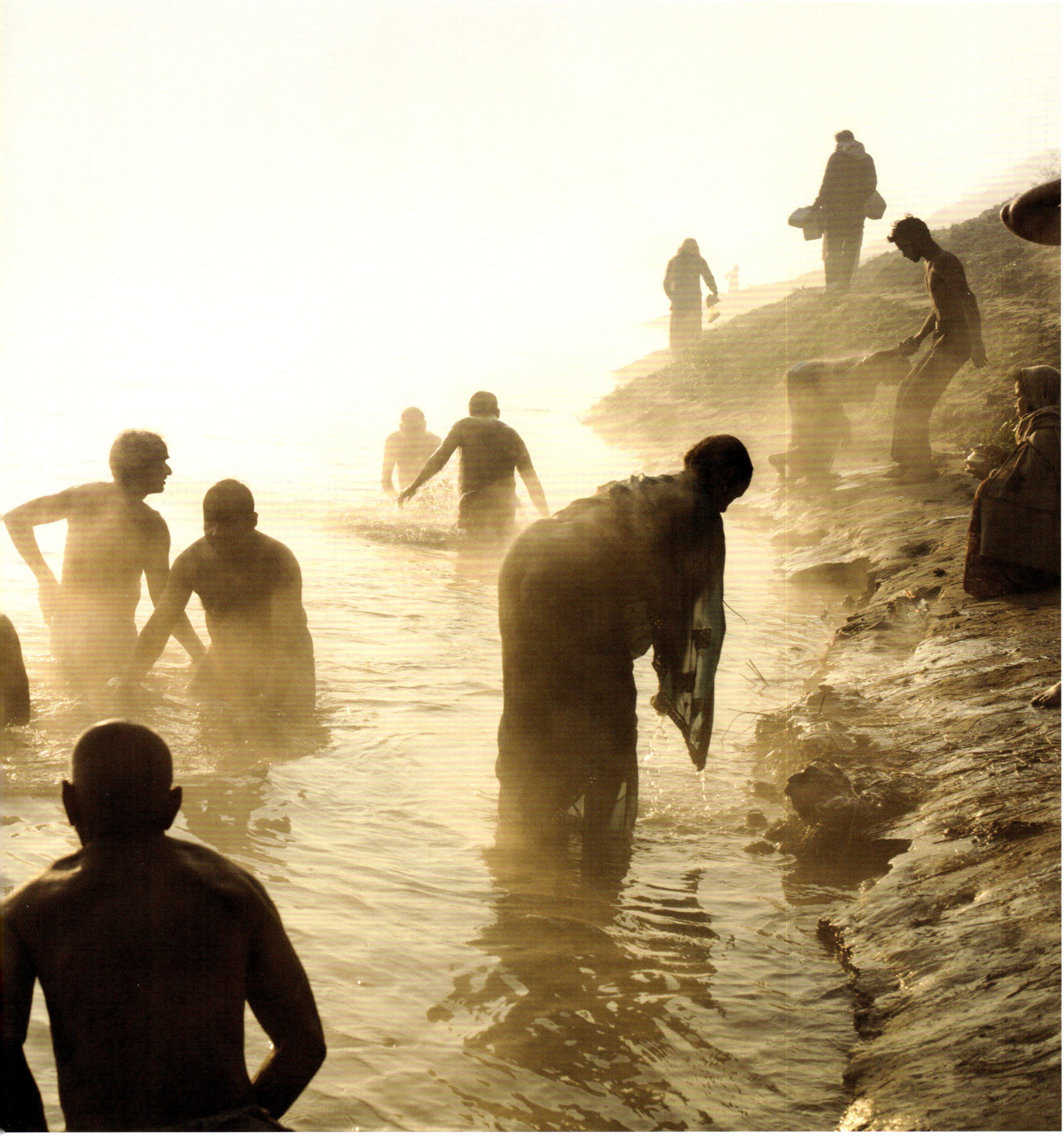

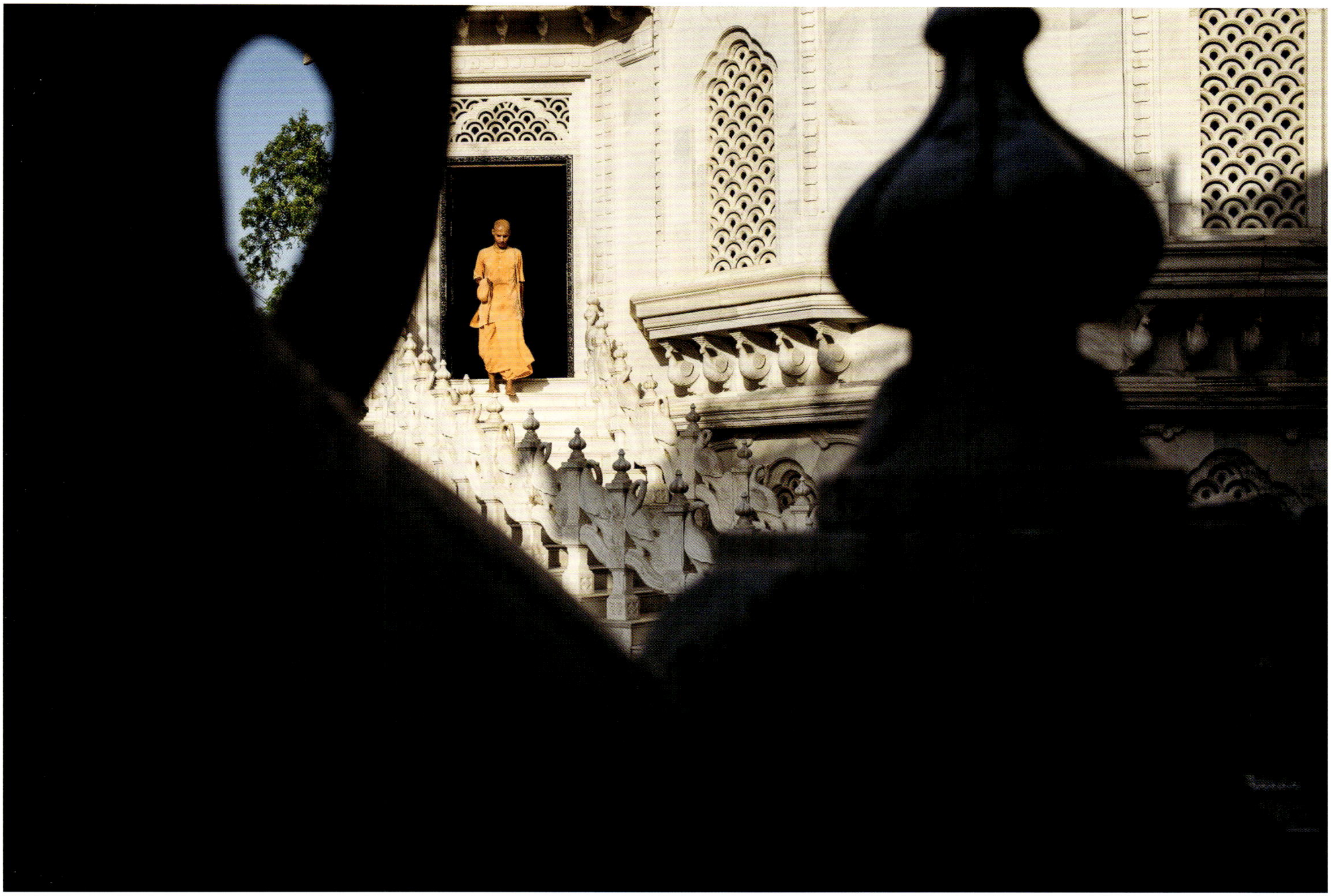

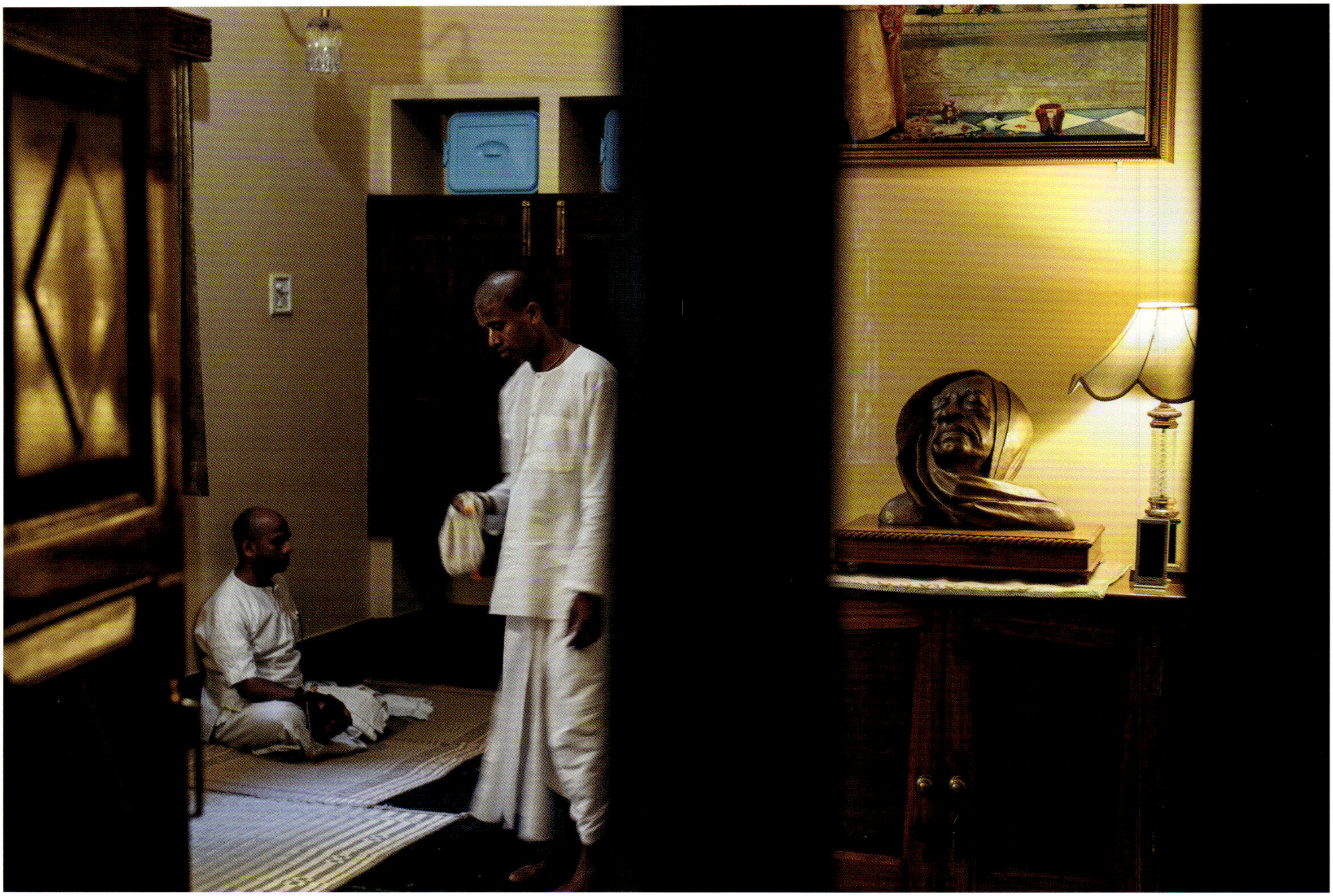

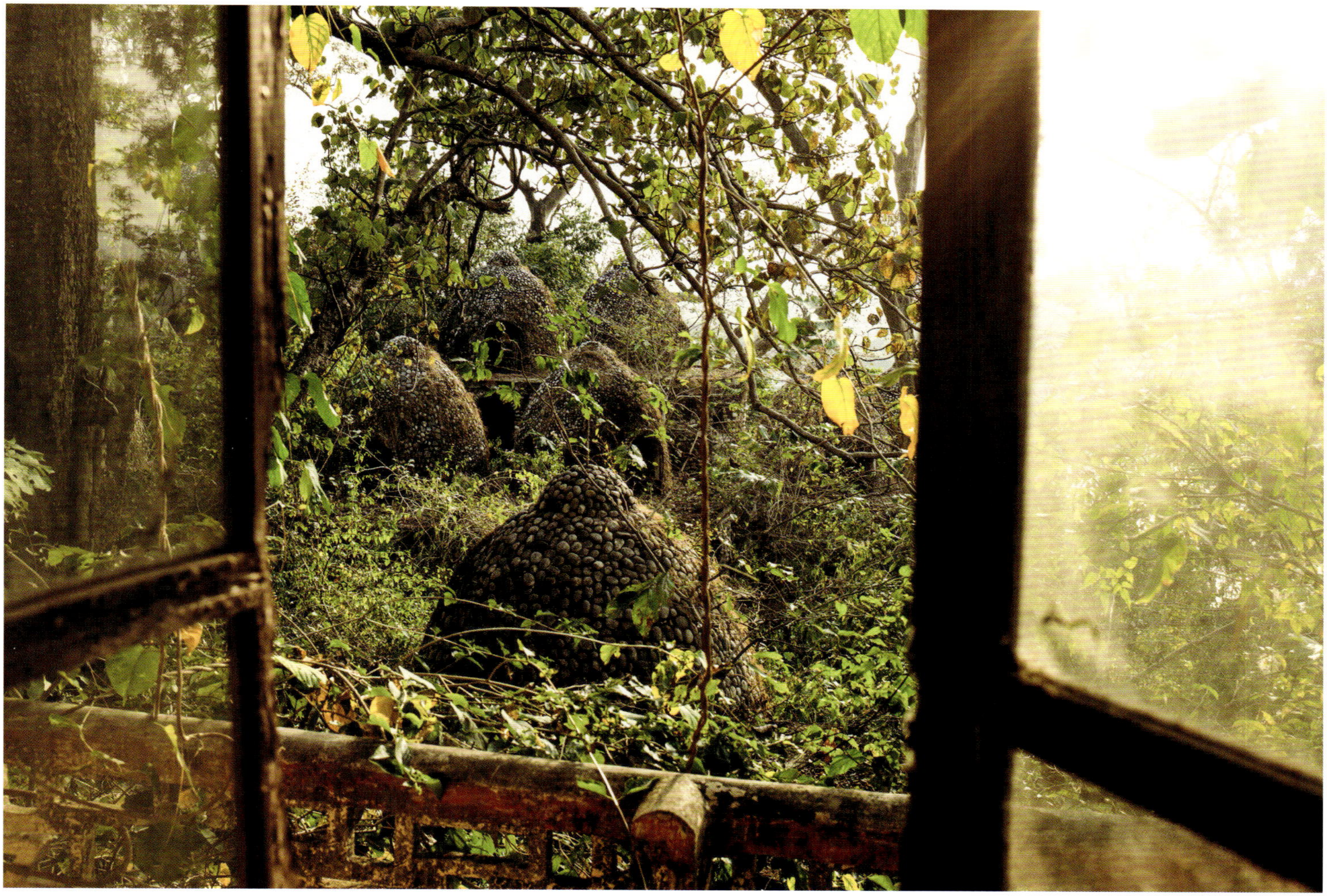

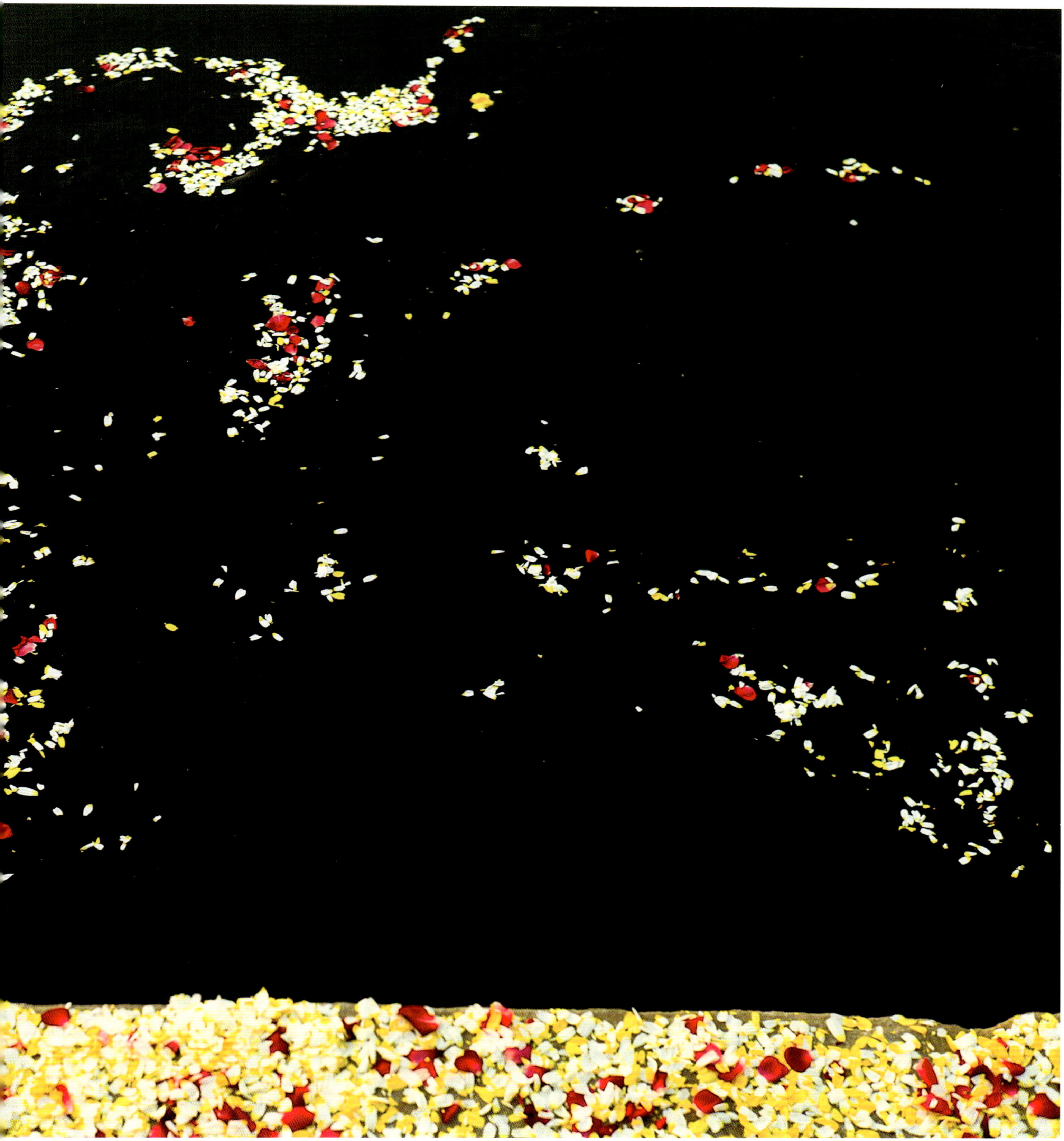

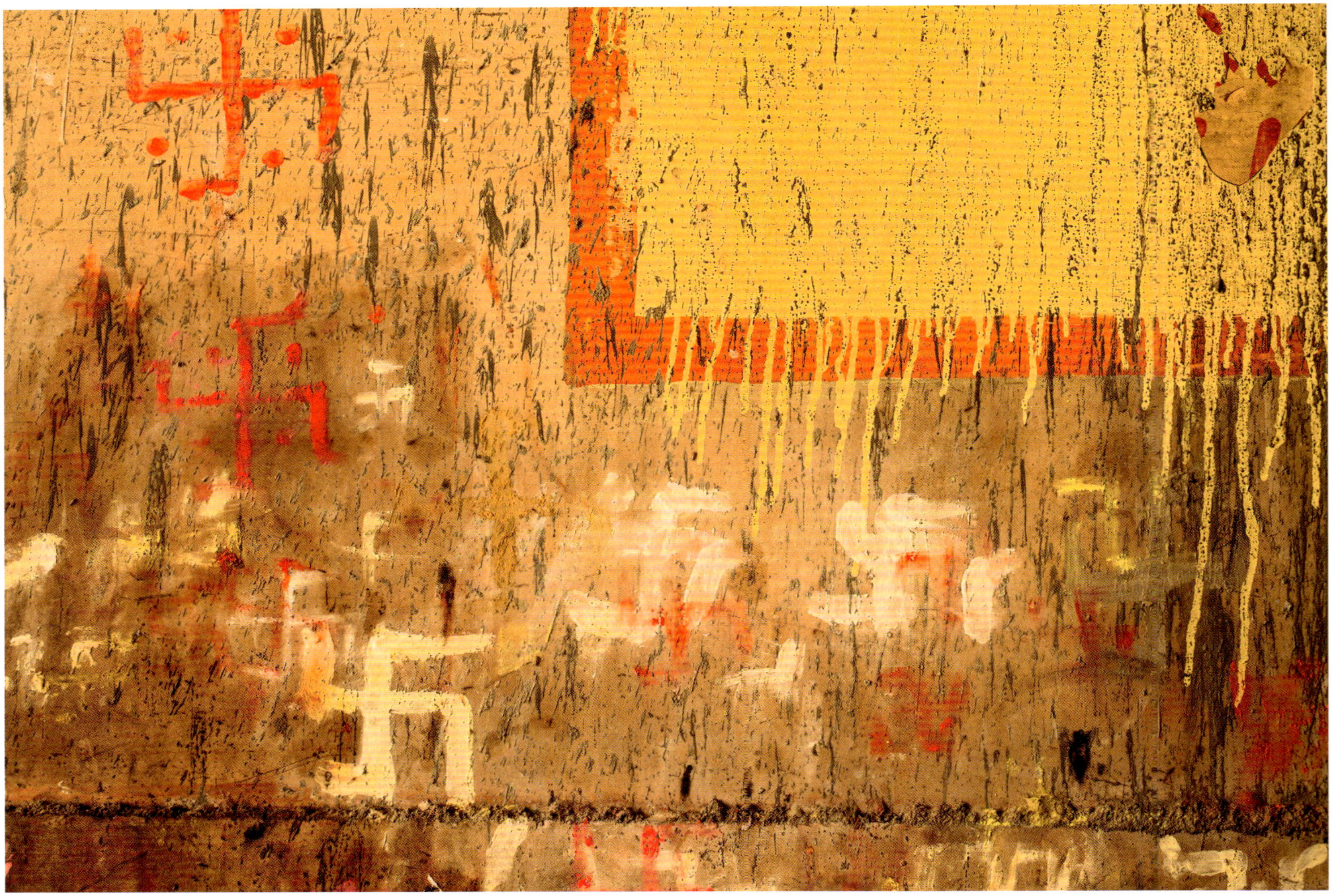

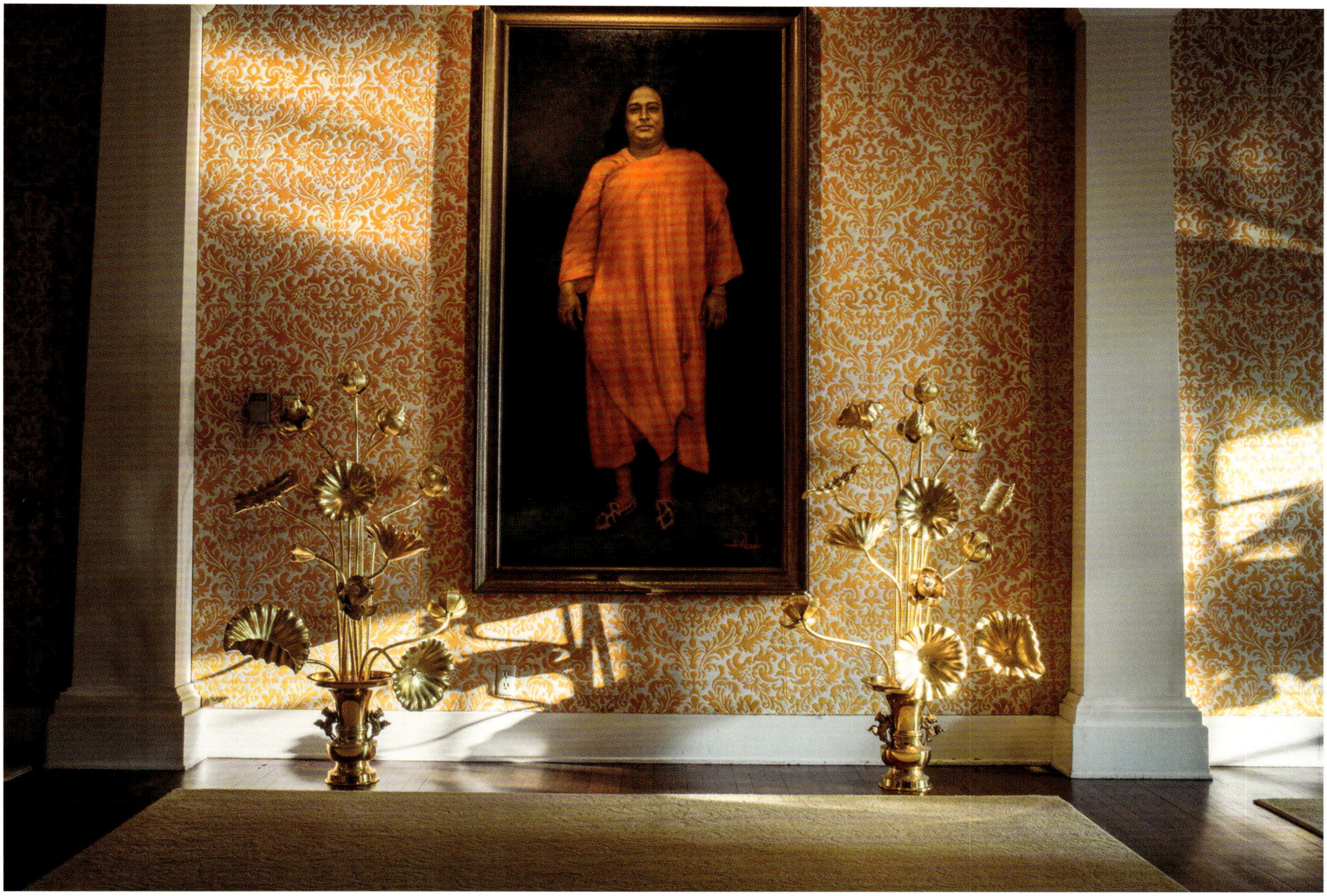

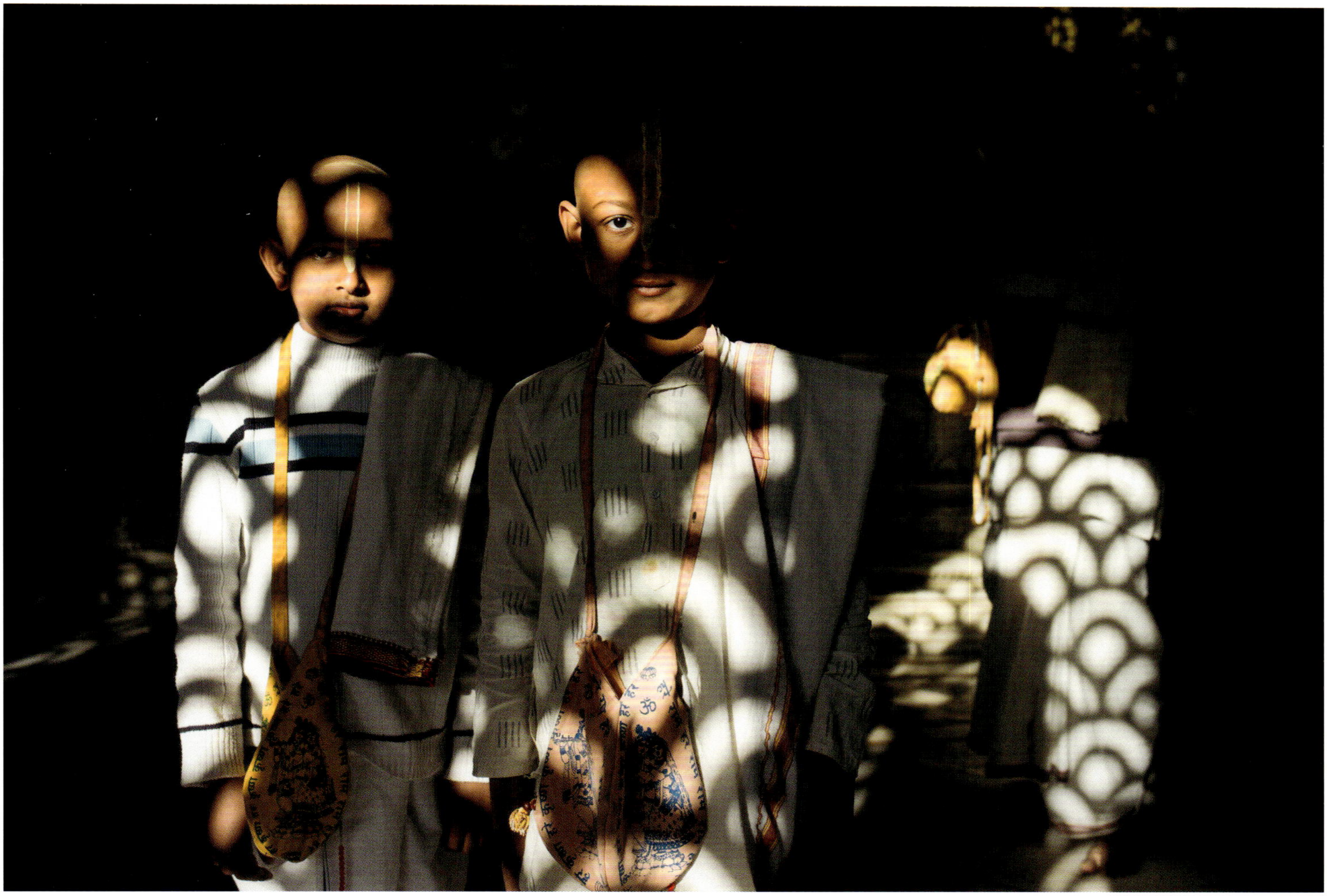

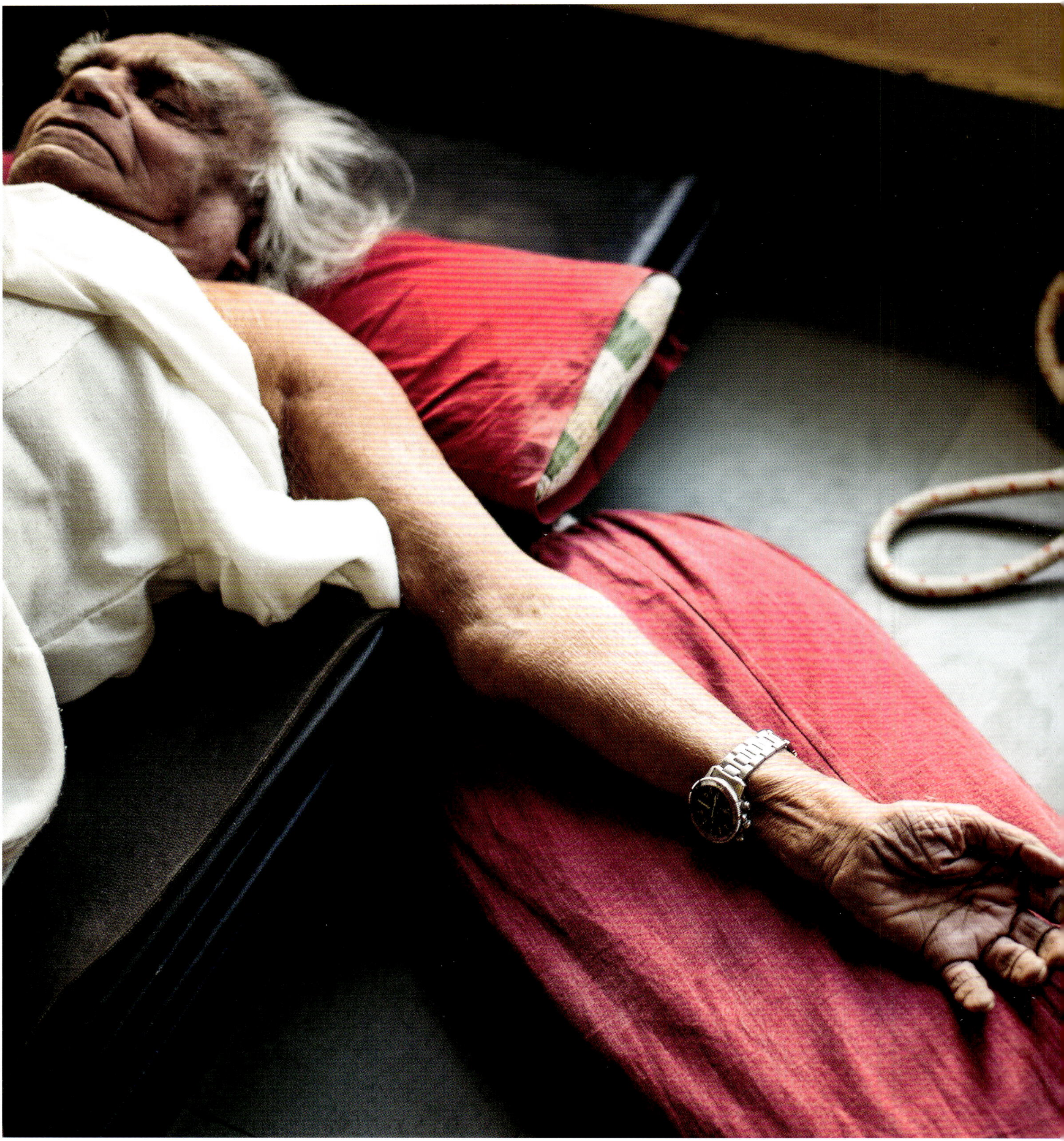

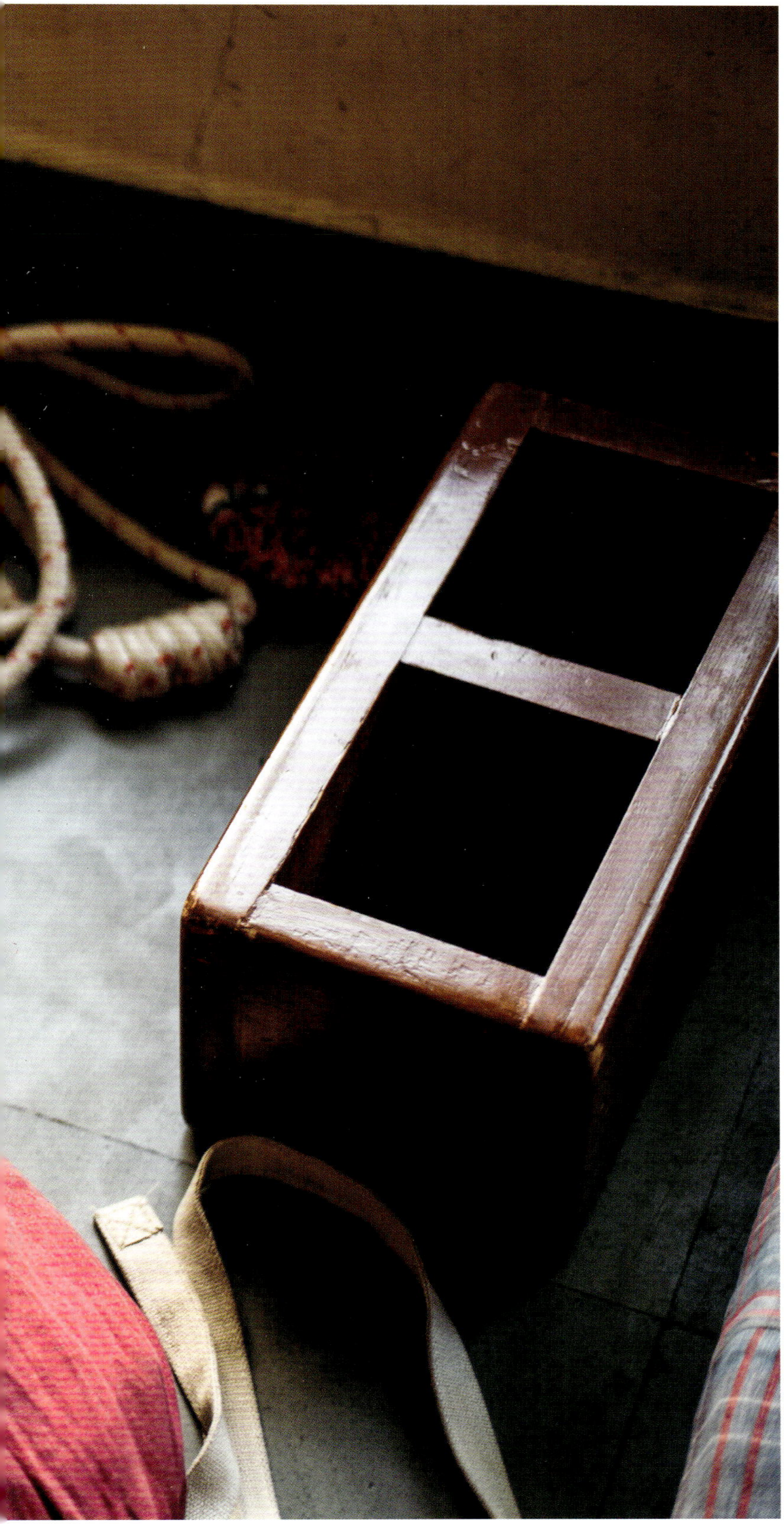

Afterword

Surrounded by yogis, I am present. It is happening. All around me, consciousness shifts and transforms. While many see physical exercise or people sitting still in a room, that is merely the surface. There is something profound occurring before my lens.

On a purely physiological level, we know the effect of a pose: muscles are working, glands are activated, and organs are squeezed. *Prana*, or life force, circulates, replenishing with every breath. The brain is stimulated and cleared. With each movement, essential messages are communicated.

Practiced on a regular basis, with intention, these superficial benefits alone will change one's life. Yet the body is but a vehicle, the container through which yoga is known. There are vast resources within us that are unacknowledged and unexplored.

Each of us has immense wisdom, here and now, waiting to be tapped. Through the subtle work of *sadhana* (daily practice), clarity, intuition, and peace are revealed. We begin to grasp our true depths, to see the other as our self, to know the interconnected nature of reality.

Yoga becomes an experience of Union.

Radhanath Swami, a monk in the Krishna-bhakti lineage, put it to me this way, "The Sanskrit word *yoga* means to reconnect with our eternal essence. And the purpose of every aspect of yoga is to create a transformation of our character, a transformation of our perception of life, and a transformation of our consciousness, from arrogance to humility, from greed to generosity, from vengeance to forgiveness, from hate to love, from agitation to peace. And ultimately, in this world, from envy to compassion. Because unless those transformations take place, unless we tap into our own spiritual essence, our true nature, there can be no real fulfillment in life."

In creating these photographs, many great saints and masters humbly welcomed me, sharing their wisdom over the years. I was invited to enter worlds I did not know existed and awakened to something true. This is my offering to yoga, for which I am eternally grateful.

Andy Richter

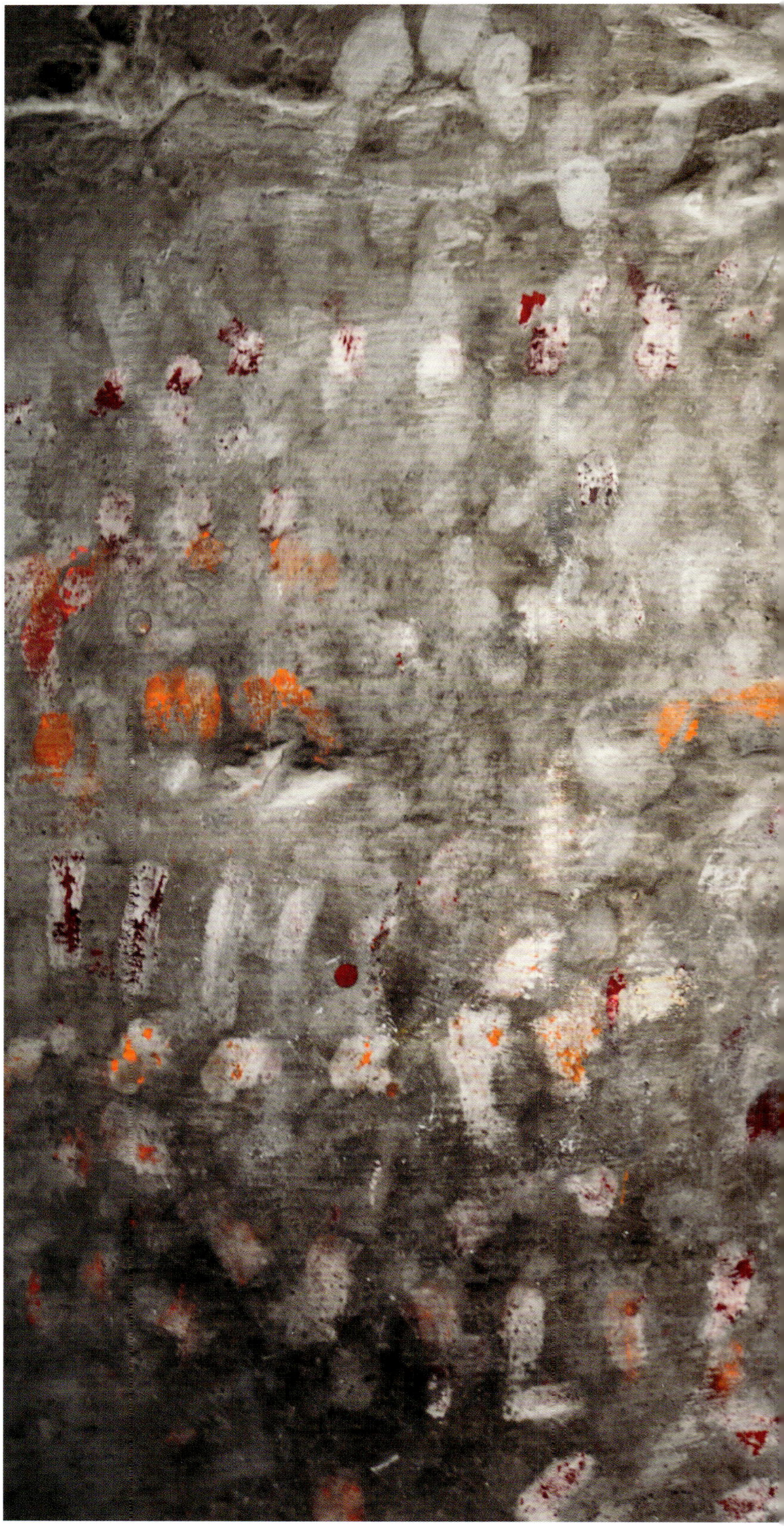

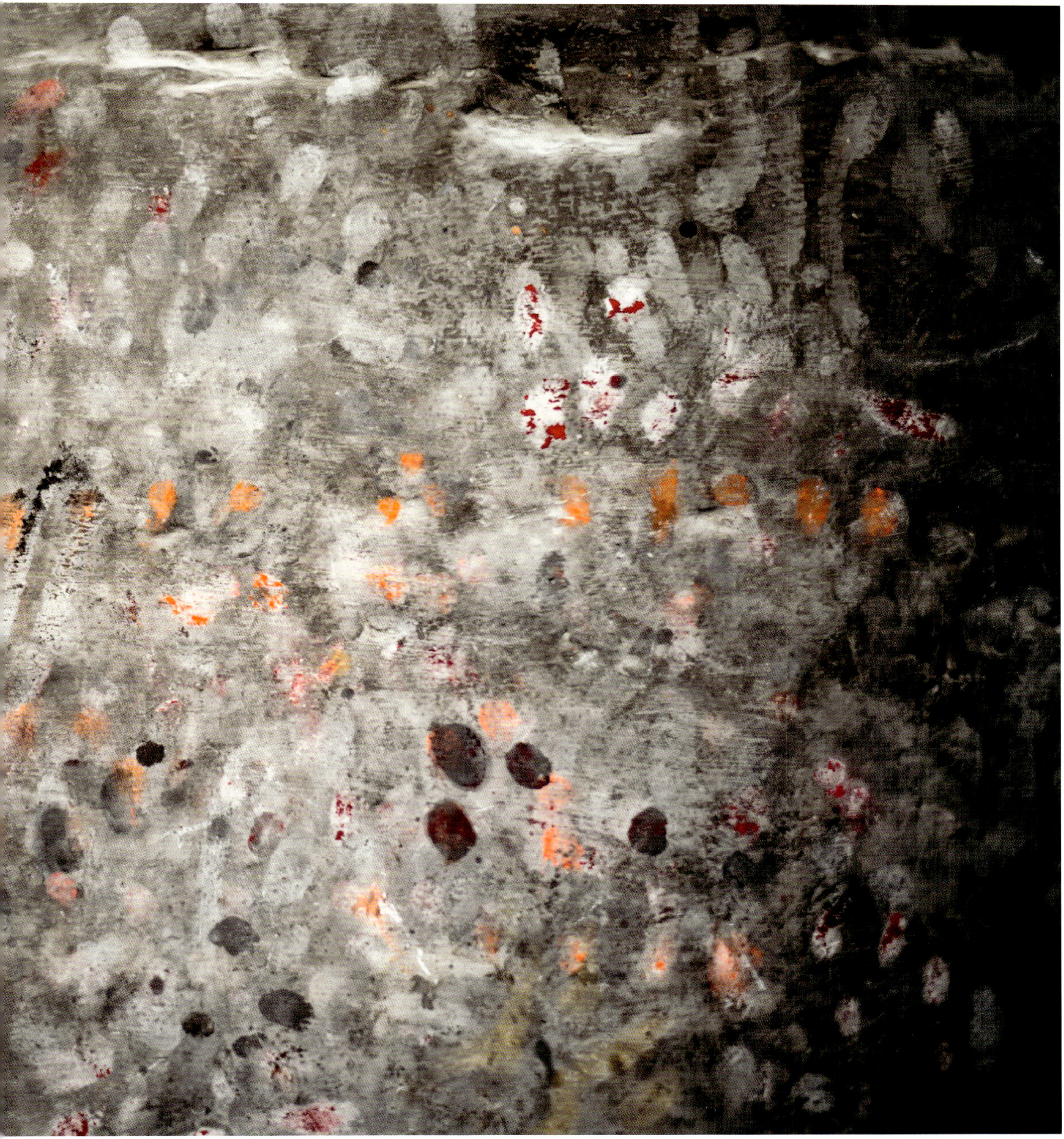

Notes on selected photographs

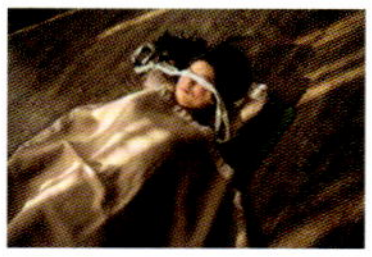

A yogini lies in *savasana* or "corpse pose," at Yogi Yoga in Beijing. The Chinese people have engaged in mind-body practices for centuries, yet the state, suspicious of activity that could undermine the collective order, has been slow to embrace yoga as a method of personal realization. Today, the official stance appears to be shifting. Mohan Bhandari, the founder of Yogi Yoga, the country's most popular chain of studios, said that yoga is growing 20% annually.

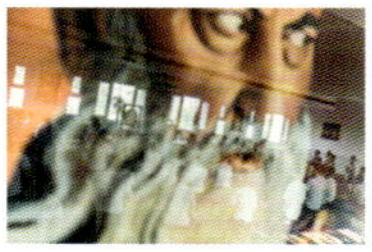

Students at Miri Piri Academy in Amritsar, India, practice Kundalini yoga in the reflection of Yogi Bhajan. In Kundalini yoga, there are thousands of *kriyas* consisting of postures, *pranayama* (breath techniques), and meditations. Kriyas are often maintained for substantial periods of time, allowing the mind to give way to the body's wisdom, to transcend ego, and to clear limiting beliefs and patterns within.

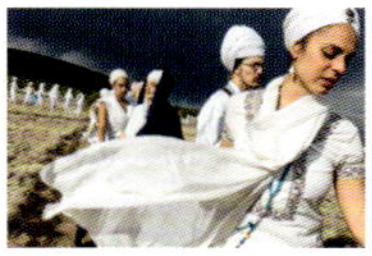

Following two and a half days of White Tantric Yoga, yogis in New Mexico take a blind walk through the arid landscape. With eyes closed, the group is led by a leader who calls out "Wahe Guru" while those following respond "Wahe Guru," an expression of ecstatic awe of the divine, sharing aloud the experience of going from darkness to light, from ignorance to true understanding.

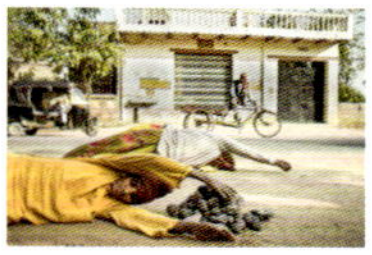

Krishna devotees prostrate during their circumambulation of Govardhan Hill, near Govardhan, India. Moving one stone her body's length with each prostration (of 108 stones), the devotee in the foreground's *parikrama*, or walk around the sacred hill, will require 12 years to complete. Her *bhakti*, or devotion to Krishna, keeps her moving forward.

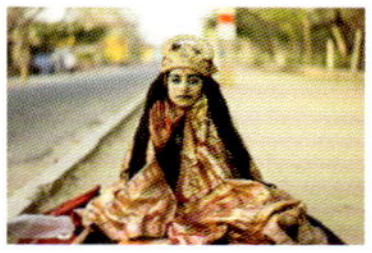

A young devotee blesses pilgrims along the Govardhan parikrama, where Krishna is believed to have spent much of his youth. According to the 10th Canto of Shrimad Bhagavatam, after Krishna protected the inhabitants of Vraj (Vrindavan) from the wrath of Indra, he counseled them to worship the holy hill through *puja* and parikrama.

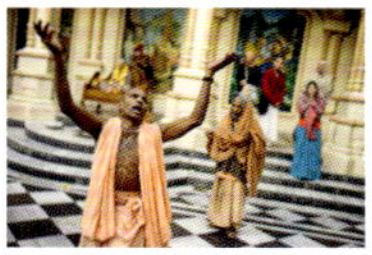

At Krishna Balaram temple in Vrindavan, India, one experiences the essence of bhakti yoga. With great love and devotion, and frequently with tears of joy in their eyes, devotees from around the globe come to the ISKCON temple to dance, sing in *kirtan*, and shower flowers upon statues of Radha and Krishna, as well as the late bhakti master and founder of Krishna consciousness, A.C. Bhaktivedanta Swami Prabhupada.

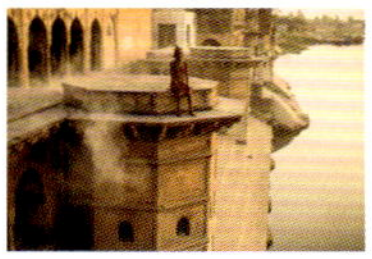

Meditation on the Yamuna River at Keshi Ghat in Vrindavan. Krishna is believed to have bathed here after killing the demon Keshi, who symbolizes pride in ones devotional practices, vanity, and ego. Bhakti yogis curtail such tendencies through chanting and humble service.

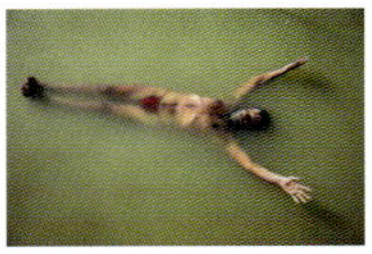

A *sadhu* practices *plavini pranayama* while floating on the Shipra River during the Kumbh Mela in Ujjain, India. In this breath exercise, the blood flows rapidly in the body, removing impurities and accumulated toxins. It is said that yogis who master this pranayama can sustain life for days without food.

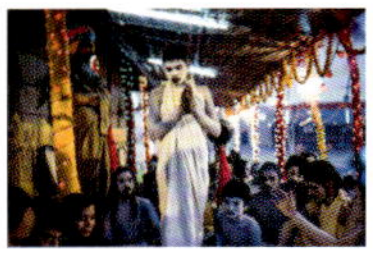

Young initiates perform puja at the Panchayati Bada Udasin Akhara during the Maha Kumbh Mela in Allahabad, India. At the confluence of India's three holy rivers—the Ganges, the Yamuna, and the mythical Saraswati—a great Hindu fair comes to life every 12 years. Drawing approximately 100 million pilgrims to Allahabad over 55 days, the Maha Kumbh is the largest human gathering on the planet. On the principal bathing days, 20 to 30 million people come to the Sangam, the holy bathing area where the rivers join, for a dip in the sacred waters.

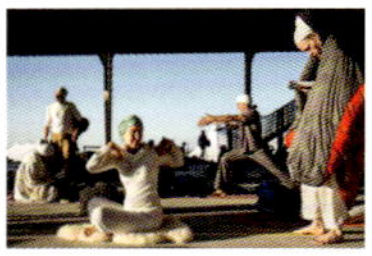

Yogis practice *asana* as the sun rises during Summer Solstice Sadhana, a yoga festival at Ram Das Puri in New Mexico. A group of singing minstrels, led by Guru Singh, walks through camp at 3 a.m. each morning encouraging all to "rise up" for morning sadhana, a two and a half hour series of meditations, mantras, and postures to begin the day. Yogi Bhajan, who brought Kundalini yoga to the West from India in 1968, taught that daily practice is essential for personal spiritual development.

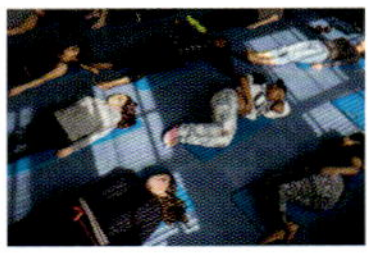

Students lay in savasana during their weekly yoga class for pregnant teens at Thomas Riley High School in Watts, California. The program is lead by Krishna Kaur and her organization, Yoga for Youth, which brings yoga and meditation to schools and youth detention centers.

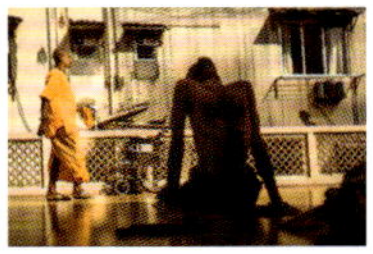

A monk in the Krishna-bhakti lineage practices *urdhva mukha svanasana* on the roof of Radha Gopinath Temple in Mumbai, India, while another devotee chants the maha mantra in walking meditation. Brahmacharis wear saffron to symbolize their renunciation and commitment to live in selfless service to others.

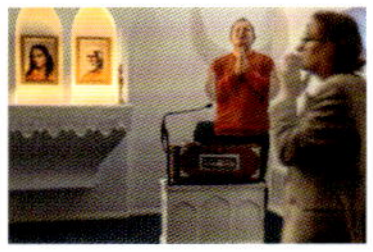

Morning invocation during a retreat at the Self-Realization Fellowship (SRF) hermitage in Encinitas, California. Paramahansa Yogananda founded the SRF in 1920 and is author of the yoga classic, *Autobiography of a Yogi*, which he wrote while living at the hermitage, which overlooks the Pacific Ocean.

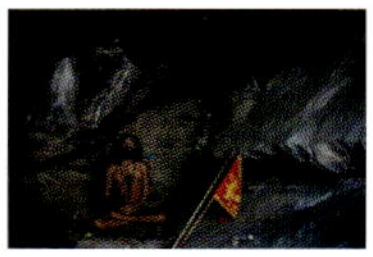

Bhandari Baba, a silent yogi for over 10 years, meditates in his cave in the foothills above Rishikesh, India. Bhandari eats plants he finds in the forest or foods visitors to bring him, primarily communicating through hand gestures. For millennia, sages and saints have come to the area for meditation and self-realization. The observation of silence, or *mauna*, allows the mind to settle and awareness to turn inward.

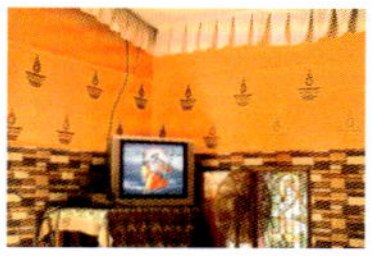

Radha and Krishna on the television at Mauni Baba Ashram near Neelkanth, India.

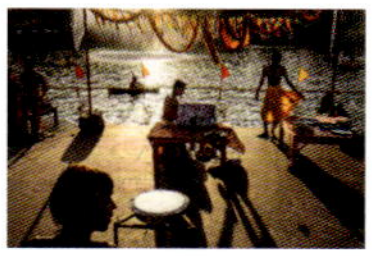

Pujaris await pilgrims bearing prayers and offerings on the Shipra River during the Kumbh Mela in Ujjain.

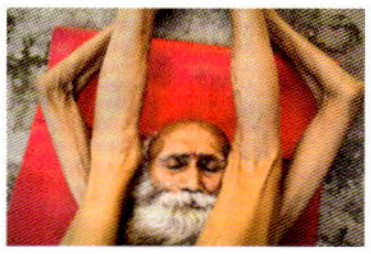

104-year-old Swami Yogananda in *supta padangusthasana* during the International Yoga Festival at Parmarth Niketan Ashram in Rishikesh. He claimed that the secret to longevity is fasting. Yogananda passed away in January of 2015.

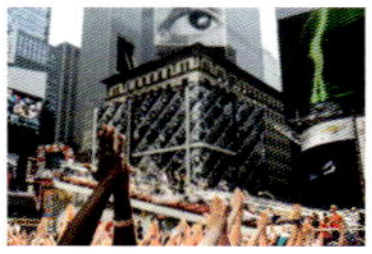

Yogis raise their hands in *virabhadrasana 1* during "Mind Over Madness" yoga in Times Square on the summer solstice. From 43rd to 48th streets along Broadway, over 8,000 came for asana and meditation during the five sessions held throughout the day. In 2014, the United Nations recognized June 21st as the "International Day of Yoga," an affirmation of yoga's ability to promote health and harmony within, among people, and with nature.

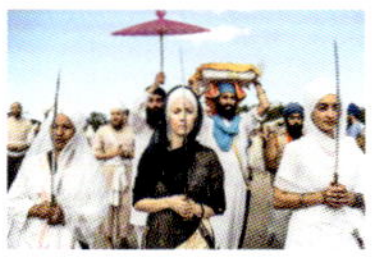

Kundalini yogis and followers of Sikh faith bring the *guru*, or holy scriptures, to the *gurdwara* (temple) in a procession known as Nagar Kirtan during Summer Solstice Sadhana.

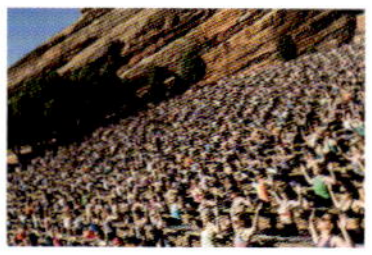

Thousands of yogis practice asana during a early morning class at Red Rocks Amphitheater near Morrison, Colorado. Approximately 3000 attended the sold out event, "Yoga on the Rocks."

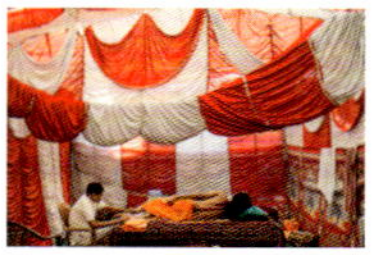

A sadhu is given a massage by a devotee at the Kumbh Mela in Ujjain.

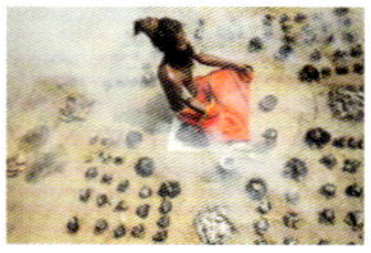

A yogi performs *panch agni tapas*, the five-fire-austerity, symbolically sacrificing himself to the fire in meditation during the Kumbh Mela in Ujjain. The intensity of the heat develops stamina and resistance in the body and helps draw the consciousness inwards. The senses become extremely sensitive and the whole body becomes like an antenna.

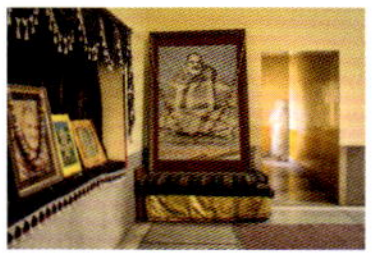

Neem Karoli Baba Ashram in Vrindavan. Guru to Steve Jobs, Ram Dass, Krishna Das, and many others, Neem Karoli Baba continues to draw devotees well after his passing in 1973. The Vrindavan ashram contains the late guru's samadhi shrine, where his body was cremated upon a sandlewood fire.

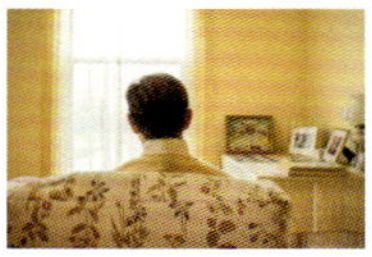

Jim Davis meditates in his Vasthu home (a traditional Hindu system of architecture), in Fairfield, Iowa. A conscious community, Fairfield has been home to Maharishi University of Management since 1974 and hosts the golden dome—the world's largest training center for practitioners of Transcendental Meditation.

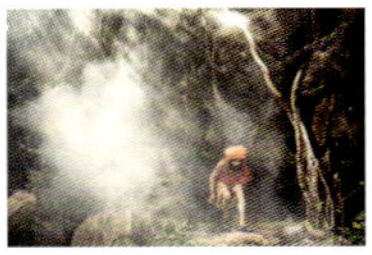

Guru Saran Das is smoked out of Mauni Baba cave while burning cow dung in the forested hills above Rishikesh. He has done his sadhana and lived in the cave for over 12 years.

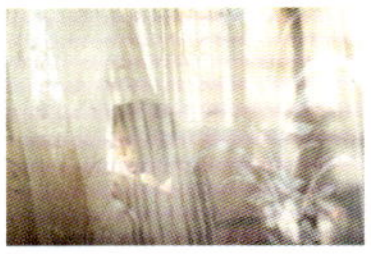

Yogis chant mantras at the close of their Ashtanga practice with Saraswathi Jois, daughter of the late yoga master Sri K. Pattabhi Jois, in Mysore, India. Saraswathi and her son Sharath, continue to teach traditional Ashtanga yoga and lead a global community of students.

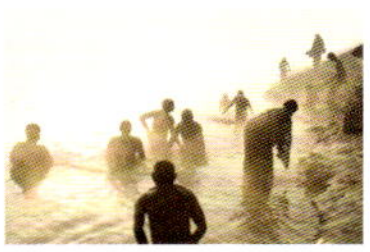

Sunrise on the Ganges River during Mauni Amavasya Snan, the primary bathing day of the Maha Kumbh Mela in Allahabad.

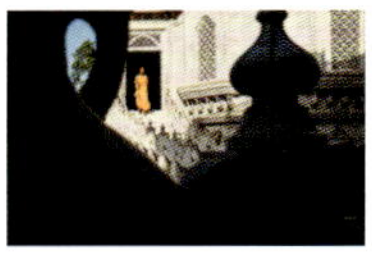

A brahmachari chants the maha mantra in walking meditation at Krishna Balaram Temple in Vrindavan. The Hare Krishna mantra has been sung continuously in kirtan 24 hours a day since 1986 at the temple.

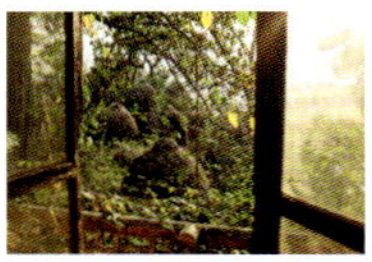

Meditation pods lie overgrown and abandoned on the banks of the Ganges River at Chaurasi Kutia Ashram, also known as "The Beatles Ashram," near Rishikesh. In 1968, the band visited Maharishi Mahesh Yogi's ashram to attend an advanced Transcendental Meditation (TM) training course. Their adoption of the Maharishi as their guru is credited by many for changing attitudes in the West about Indian spirituality and yoga.

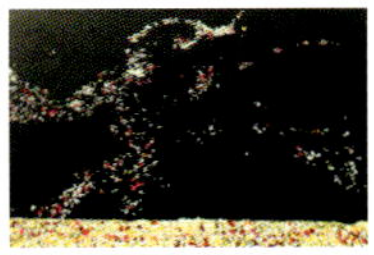

Petals of devotion flow with the Yamuna River near Keshi Ghat in Vrindavan.

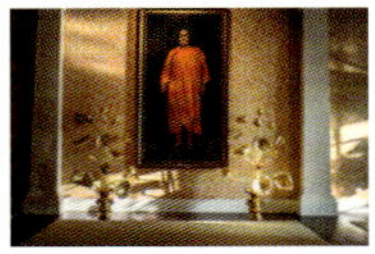

A portrait of Paramahansa Yogananda at the Self-Realization Fellowship (SRF) headquarters in Los Angeles, California. The title, *Serpent in the Wilderness*, was inspired by Yogananda's interpretation of the biblical passage John 3:13-15: "No one has ever gone into heaven except the one who came from heaven— the Son of Man. Just as Moses lifted up the snake in the wilderness, so the Son of Man must be lifted up, that everyone who believes may have eternal life in him." He suggests that "serpent" refers to Kundalini energy, or man's consciousness coiled at the base of the spine, which must be raised up for true spiritual liberation. The "wilderness" is the silence of meditation.

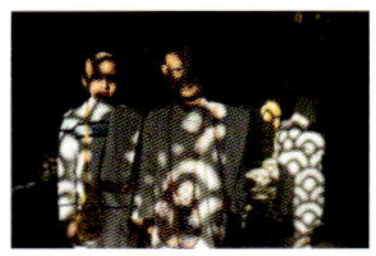

Young devotees in the Samadhi Mandir of A.C. Bhaktivedanta Swami Prabhupada at Krishna Balaram Temple in Vrindavan.

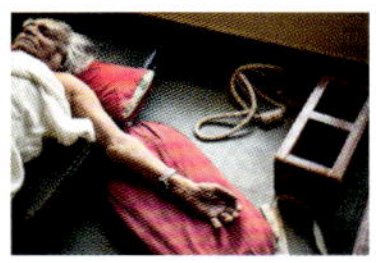

B.K.S. Iyengar in savasana at Ramamani Iyengar Memorial Yoga Institute in Pune, India. Iyengar is responsible for sharing yoga with arguably more human beings than any other person in history. Traditionally, yoga was passed directly from guru to student in an intimate relationship; Iyengar brought yoga to a classroom context, changing its trajectory forever. An honor to photograph, Iyengar passed away on August 20, 2014. Up to his 95th year, he practiced asana daily and shared his vast knowledge and experience with his students.

Acknowledgements

Exploring yoga has enriched my life in so many ways. This book was brought into being with the support of many people: family and friends, photographers, editors, curators, and a global community of yogis, past and present. I held the intention and followed it with action, and the doors began to open.

First, I would like to thank Alexa Becker and Klaus Kehrer for seeing the potential in this project and offering to make a book together. I am grateful to have such a talented team of collaborators at Kehrer Verlag, including Martin Lutz, René Henoch, Katharina Stumpf, Andreas Schubert, Barbara Karpf, and Katharina Windfuhr. A special thank you to Bonnie Briant who realized the initial design and laid a solid foundation for the book's concept and final form. I also would like to acknowledge Ethan Jones for his beautiful prints and assistance in bringing the photographs to life on paper. Thank you Ann Kirby McGill, Melissa Rivard, Jonathan Blaustein, and Tasha Eichenseher for your suggestions and keen editing.

I greatly appreciate the guidance of Alex Webb and Rebecca Norris Webb, whose insight helped me distill the work down to its essence and find a rhythm and flow in the sequence. I would also like to acknowledge the late Mary Ellen Mark for her support and generosity over the years. Many thanks to my friends and peers in the photography community who helped make this book a reality, in particular Scott B. Davis, Elizabeth Krist, Andrew Fedynak, Elizabeth Avedon, Joshua Farr, Sharon Lavier O'Keefe, Mark Davis, Marin Stefani, and my first photography teacher, Lester Hughes-Seamans. I am grateful to live in a place that supports the arts, and would specifically like to thank the Minnesota State Arts Board for supporting my work.

There are many yogis who helped illuminate the way forward; without them, this book would not exist, and the world would be a darker place. I would like to acknowledge the following for their presence and selfless service to humanity: the late B.K.S. Iyengar, Radhanath Swami, Sadhvi Bhagawati Saraswati, Erich Shiffmann, Saraswathi Jois, Swami Ramdev, Acharya Balkrishna, Matthew Sanford, Dharma Mittra, Swami Laxman Das, Krishna Kaur, Guru Jagat, Harijwan, Adarsh Kaur Khalsa, Jugat Guru Singh Khalsa, Mohan Bhandari, Shiva Das, Swami Chandra Giri, Swami Laxman Das Jaya, Swami Sarvadevananda, A.C. Bhaktivaibhava Swami, Neeraj Nautiyal, Bhandari Baba, Swami Nardanand, Ken Chawkin, Nirmal Lumpkin, Deepika Mehta, Eddie Stern, Dr. Fred Travis, Matthew Portwood, Jumpei Kontani, Brent Horning, Mark Stephens, and Brenda Flemming.

This book would not have been possible without the generous support of the following individuals and families: Abhai Raj and Sat Purkh Khalsa, Guillermo Treviño B., Norma Deschamps, the Gralton family, Sydney Holly, Joel Larson, Tara Daily, James and Diane Davis, R.J. Kern, Anja Bruehling, Laura Salazar, Peter Hunner, and the Reece family.

Most importantly, I would like to thank my family for their encouragement and steadfast support, especially my brothers Peter and Jesse, and my mother and late father, whose love has been with me from the beginning. Dad, I wish I could share these photographs and this moment with you. I offer my deepest gratitude to my wife and partner in life, Selma—a loving mother and talented photographer, my most trusted editor and friend. Thank you for helping to realize this dream.

This book is dedicated to Julien, our joyous newborn son, who has brought so many blessings into our life. May you know your Self.

Your own Self-Realization
is the greatest service you can
render the world.

Ramana Maharshi

Design: Bonnie Briant, Andy Richter, and Kehrer Design Heidelberg (Martin Lutz) **Image Processing**: Kehrer Design Heidelberg (René Henoch) **Copy Editing**: Ann Kirby McGill **Proofreading**: Anthony Santoro **Production**: Kehrer Design Heidelberg (Andreas Schubert)

Cover Photograph: Manasi Ganga Abstraction, Govardhan, India, 2016.

Printed and bound in Germany
ISBN 978-3-86828- 845-2

Kehrer Heidelberg Berlin
www.kehrerverlag.com